ADHD ORGANIZING AND CLEANING SOLUTIONS

UNLOCK THE POWER OF THE 5-MINUTE TASK
TO AVOID STRESS AND OVERWHELM, BEAT
PROCRASTINATION AND TRANSFORM YOUR
HOME INTO A CLUTTER-FREE ZONE

CAROLINE SINGER

CONTENTS

INTRODUCTION

The best way to get something done is to begin.

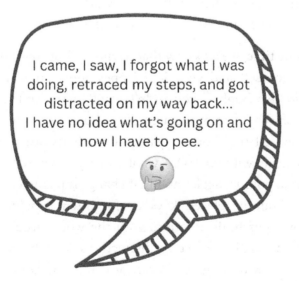

Have you ever put a load of laundry into the dryer and forgotten to switch it on? The clothes sit there patiently for a week before you open the dryer again, and you are reunited with a pile of smelly, damp laundry. Or have you ever missed an important event at your child's school, even though you reminded yourself that morning? Maybe you have a 'doom pile' of unsorted clutter staring accusingly at you in every room, unwashed dishes piled up in the sink, a bursting closet that you would rather not open and an inbox of unread emails that is starting to stress you out? This is a daily reality for many people with ADHD, for whom the desire to organize clashes with the brain's unique wiring.

First things first – this does NOT make you a bad person. We can be kind, happy, generous, loving and successful human beings without being great at doing the dishes or keeping the living room tidy. How you organize your life and care for your home is not a reflection of your character and your worth. You don't have to do it all, and you certainly don't have to do it all in one go.

At the same time, we all know that having a clean and tidy house is a gift to yourself and your loved ones, and you wouldn't have purchased this book if you didn't want to try and make some changes or see an improvement. This book was born from the realization that traditional organizing methods often don't work for individuals with ADHD. I want to let you know that you are not alone in your struggles and that change *is* possible, because it's not just about misplaced keys or forgotten appointments; it's about how your brain interacts with the world around you in a uniquely challenging dance of distractions. This book is here to provide you with practical strategies and empathetic support, tailored to your unique needs.

In this book, I am going to explain different ways of helping you manage and organize your life. One of the main focuses will be the 5-minute task technique, a strategy developed specifically to help adults with ADHD. In essence, this means breaking down cleaning, organizing and decluttering tasks into manageable 5-minute chunks. It's about making the process so simple and quick that starting doesn't seem daunting, and finishing feels achievable. This technique has the potential to transform your daily life, making it more manageable and less stressful.

The beauty of these 5-minute strategies is their transformative power. Not only can they help you create a clutter-free environment, but they also reduce stress, enhance your mental health, and improve your overall quality of life.

Celebrating small victories and making step-by-step progress is at the heart of this approach, reinforcing that every minute spent organizing moves you closer to a calmer, more controlled environment.

This book isn't about achieving a picture-perfect home. That's absolutely not where we are coming from and not what we are looking for. As K.C. Davis says, "no-one ever lays on their deathbed wishing they'd cleaned the bathroom more." It's about making small, realistic, sustainable changes that improve our day-to-day life and our sense of being able to manage. It's perfectly okay if things aren't immaculate. What matters is the progress we make each time we try, and the habits we develop along the way. Aiming for 'good enough' really and truly *is* good enough!

Throughout this guide, you'll find a whole range of practical decluttering and cleaning strategies that will help you make a start on different areas of your home, taking each task step-by-step to avoid overwhelm. There's also deep dives into topics such as digital decluttering, the art of the brain dump for clearing your mind, great tips for grocery shopping and meal planning, and much more.

This book is written specifically with the ADHD brain in mind: chapters and paragraphs are kept short so that you don't get bogged down with too much text. There's lots of bullet points and lists for quick reference, and an empathetic yet practical approach that I really hope will resonate with you. The book covers three broad themes: organization, decluttering and cleaning. Each chapter is more or less self-contained, so if you want, you can zoom straight to the chapters that you need the most. The speech bubbles you will find in each chapter are real-life quotes from people just like you, who have trodden this path too, and found solutions that really work. (There are also a few ADHD memes scattered about to make you smile!)

Coming from a place of deep empathy and understanding of the ADHD brain, this book aims to be a supportive companion on your journey. There are lots of books out there on organization, and some systems have become world-famous. Not so many books have been written with the individual with ADHD in mind. Everyone is looking for that one specific book that speaks to their soul. I hope with all my heart that this book will speak to yours. As we move forward, remember this: every small step you take is a victory. With each task done, you are not just organizing your space, but reclaiming your life. Let's begin this journey together, one small step at a time.

CHAPTER 1
UNDERSTANDING ADHD
AND ORGANIZATION

ADHD is knowing you have a
deadline, wasting time for eight
hours, then neglecting all your
body's basic needs until it's
done.

L et's play a little game of Myth-Busters, ADHD style. You've probably heard it all before: "People with ADHD just need to try harder," or "They're just using ADHD as an excuse to be lazy." Sound familiar? Let's set the record straight. ADHD isn't a warehouse for excuses, and it certainly isn't a one-size-fits-all disorder, especially when it comes to organization. Understanding these myths and the reality of ADHD is like finding the right pair of glasses—suddenly, everything comes into focus.

Myth vs. Reality

First off, the biggie: the myth that individuals with ADHD are simply lazy or unmotivated. Here's the truth—ADHD involves various executive function impairments, including challenges with activation, effort, and memory. This means tasks that require organization can sometimes feel like assembling a thousand-piece puzzle with no reference image. Not exactly a lazy Sunday afternoon activity! This isn't a lack of will or effort; it's a neurological detour. Recognizing this helps in framing ADHD not as a deficit of character but as a different way of brain functioning that requires different strategies, fostering a more empathetic understanding of the challenges individuals with ADHD face with organization.

Now, let's talk about the common perception that people with ADHD are always disorganized. While it's true that many struggle with traditional organization, it doesn't mean they are incapable of order. Instead, their organization often looks different. It might be a workspace that looks chaotic to others but makes perfect sense to the person using it. It's the organized chaos where creativity and brilliance often thrive.

The ADHD Brain and Organization: Unveiling the Connection

The brain of an individual with ADHD isn't just a whirlwind of thoughts; it's a complex ecosystem where neurotransmitters like dopamine play a pivotal role. Typically, ADHD is marked by an underproduction of dopamine, which affects the brain's executive functions, such as focus, memory, and organizational skills. Dopamine is like the brain's motivational speaker, encouraging you to finish tasks and find pleasure in completing them. When there's a shortage, as often seen in ADHD, staying on task and keeping things organized isn't just difficult—it can feel nearly impossible.

On top of that, the ADHD brain is often deficient in a lesser-known neurotransmitter called norepinephrine, which typically helps to fire up and maintain your attention and keep you alert and on-task.

This unique wiring significantly impacts how time is perceived. For many with ADHD, the concept of time is not linear but rather a fluid, expansive entity. This can result in a skewed perception of how long tasks really take, leading to procrastination or last-minute rushes. Ever thought you had plenty of time to get ready and leave the house, only to end up sprinting to your appointment? That's your ADHD brain playing tricks with time.

The Role of Dopamine and Norepinephrine

Knowing more about the role of dopamine and norepinephrine in the ADHD brain is vital in helping to understand the challenges a person with ADHD faces every day. Dopamine is often called the 'reward chemical' in our brain, helping us with motivation and completing a task in the hope of achieving a reward. Reduced dopamine in the ADHD brain means that not all tasks are rewarding enough to sustain attention. This is why mundane jobs like filing papers or tidying your desk can feel unappealing, if not torturous.

But dopamine isn't just about pleasure; it's also essential for attention and cognitive control. For someone with ADHD, the lack of dopamine means that you are far more easily distracted while writing that report, and have a hard time ignoring every little thing that's going on around you.

Thirdly, dopamine affects executive functioning, which controls the planning, problem-solving, and decision-making aspects of life. This is why it's sometimes hard to make plans or decide which items of clutter to get rid of and which to keep, or which emails to delete and which to file.

Norepinephrine plays a part in our 'fight or flight' response, our attention regulation and our state of alertness. But it isn't just about feeling alert; it's also about staying focused on a task. A lack of norepinephrine in the ADHD brain can lead to an inability to sustain attention, which is why you might start a job but get bored very quickly. It controls our impulsiveness and hyperactivity, explaining why we sometimes fail to think before we speak. If your sleep patterns are disrupted and you have trouble sleeping at night, you can also blame this on an imbalance of norepinephrine.

Understanding Overwhelm

Why do traditional organizing methods often hit a wall when it comes to ADHD? Imagine walking into a room filled with clattering noises from every direction. That's how a typical organizing strategy can feel to someone with ADHD. Faced with a massive pile of stuff that you need to "sort, purge, organize" can quickly become overwhelming, not because the steps are complex, but because deciding what fits into these categories requires a level of decision-making that can be taxing on the ADHD brain. This often leads to what's known as analysis paralysis, where the decision-making process itself becomes a formidable barrier.

Traditional methods also fail to account for the ADHD brain's need for immediate rewards and feedback. Long-term goals are great, but when your dopamine-driven brain is screaming for a quick win, it's easy to see why a six-hour deep-cleaning session on a Saturday doesn't sound appealing. This is why breaking jobs into smaller, more manageable 'mini-tasks' can be so helpful, providing frequent doses of accomplishment and reducing the feeling of being overwhelmed.

So, now we know more, how do we make these everyday tasks more dopamine- and norepinephrine-friendly? The trick lies in making each job quick and rewarding. You don't have time to get bored or distracted, and at the end, you will be rewarded with a sense of achievement – a small victory that produces a hit of the all-important dopamine. It's really the concept of gamification, where even the most tedious task can become a mini-challenge with immediate rewards—and the best part is that you get to choose the task, the time and the reward.

Embracing Neurodiversity

If there's one thing to take away from this, it's that different doesn't mean deficient. The ADHD brain has its superpowers—hyperfocus, creativity, and the ability to think outside traditional frameworks. Embracing these strengths means shifting away from a deficit-focused view and moving towards a strengths-based organizational approach. It's about turning what might seem like quirks into qualities.

In the realm of neurodiversity, understanding that each brain has its unique wiring and preferences highlights the importance of personalized strategies in organization. What works for one person might not work for another, and that's perfectly okay. This customized approach respects and leverages individual differences for better, more sustainable organizational habits.

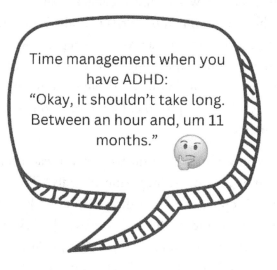

CHAPTER 2
FINDING AN ORGANIZATION SYSTEM THAT WORKS FOR YOU

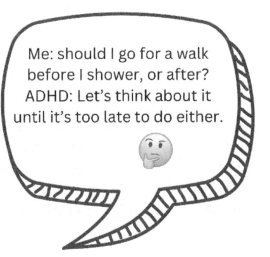

The constant buzz of ideas, obligations, deadlines and to-dos that whirl around our brain can make it hard to keep track of everything that we need to do each day. It usually doesn't take long after the first cup of coffee in the morning for the demands of the day to start invading our brain, rapidly becoming a chaotic whirlwind of competing tasks that can create strong feelings of stress and overwhelm. This is why it's vital to give yourself the gift of an organizational system – a framework to help you manage the myriad things you have to do just to keep your head above water. So, before we get down to the nitty-gritty of decluttering and cleaning, let's focus on creating an organization system that works for you.

So, what exactly is an organizational system? Put simply, it's a method to help you keep track of all the various tasks, information, responsibilities, dates and deadlines in your life, so that you can see what needs to be done and where you are heading. It can significantly reduce the clutter and confusion of your mental to-do list.

This can be as simple as telling yourself you are going to do the laundry every Tuesday and Saturday, or buying a family planner so that everyone in the household can see what is happening in the week ahead. There are many different systems, tools and techniques out there, so you can pick and choose what works best for you.

Creating a Personalized ADHD-Friendly Organization Plan

The journey of creating an organization system begins with a clear understanding of your goals and challenges. So, first things first, let's take stock of where you are now. This is absolutely not about judging or criticizing yourself for what hasn't been done; it's about understanding your starting point. What areas of your life feel most chaotic? Is it managing the household chores, dealing with work deadlines, keeping track of all those appointments and commitments, sticking to a daily routine or simply remembering to take your medication on time each day?

Next, reflect on what you want to achieve. Are you aiming for a pristine kitchen with no utensil out of place, or are you looking for a more manageable level of order that keeps the house clean and liveable without the stress of total chaos? Think about setting realistic, achievable goals. Start small and build up gradually.

Thirdly, try to identify what kind of ADHD mind you have and what organizational style will work for you. In this chapter and the following one, you will find an array of suggestions, techniques and tools you can experiment with. By understanding your challenges and goals and identifying your style, you can tailor your organizing plan to fit exactly what you need, making it more likely that you'll stick to it and actually enjoy the benefits. The key here is to work out your priorities and observe how different environments and systems affect your productivity and mood, without judgment or self-criticism.

So, let's get started. When you have a few minutes to spare, grab a notebook and pen and write down the answers to the following questions. There are no right or wrong answers; it's all about finding out what resonates with you and what comes to mind. This should help you feel clearer about how to move on and decide which organizational methods will feel less like a chore and more like a natural extension of your mind.

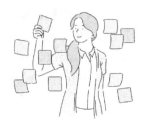

20 QUESTIONS

To help you find an organizing system that works for you

- ☐ What are your main challenges with organization?
- ☐ How does disorganization impact your daily life and well-being?
- ☐ What do you most want to change?
- ☐ In what areas of your life do you feel most disorganized ?
- ☐ What are your priority tasks?
- ☐ What have you already tried that works?
- ☐ What are your main goals for getting organized?
- ☐ Do you feel motivated by long-term goals or short-term wins?
- ☐ Do you respond well to visual prompts eg labels & color-coding?
- ☐ Are you more detail-oriented or a big-picture thinker?
- ☐ What part of your home is currently the most organized, and why?
- ☐ What are the biggest obstacles to getting organized for you?
- ☐ How much time can you devote to an organizational system?
- ☐ When do you feel most productive during the day?
- ☐ What feels most overwhelming to you?
- ☐ How do you usually prioritize your tasks?
- ☐ Do you have a budget for organizational tools and resources?
- ☐ Do you prefer digital apps, or more physical tools eg planners?
- ☐ Do you have support from others when it comes to organizing?
- ☐ Are there any tools or resources you would like to try?

These questions are intended to spark reflection and insight, guiding you towards an organizational system that suits your lifestyle and your unique needs. Start by identifying what works for you—what captures your attention, what makes you feel motivated, and what calms your anxiety. It could be as simple as organizing your books by color because it pleases your eye and inspires you to keep things neat. Or creating a schedule of chores for the whole family to follow. Perhaps you find that setting timers with different ringtones for various types of tasks helps keep you on track. The idea is to experiment with different techniques, tweak them, combine them, and invent new ones until you find a system that feels tailor-made for you.

Once you have a clearer idea of what kind of organization methods work best for you, we'll dive deeper into the different preferences and challenges you may have in the following chapters. As you go through this book, it's a good idea to make a note of the names of any new ideas and tools you might like to try.

CHAPTER 3

CREATING A PERSONALIZED, ADHD-FRIENDLY ORGANIZATION PLAN

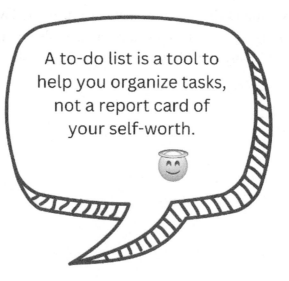

A to-do list is a tool to help you organize tasks, not a report card of your self-worth. 😇

Strategies For the Visual Thinker - Using Imagery and Color Coding

For those who think in pictures or remember things better when they are demonstrated, creating visual systems and reminders can be very helpful. Let's start with color coding, a deceptively simple yet effective tool. Imagine your filing system or wardrobe organized by color. Not only does it make finding things easier, but it also turns your space into a visually appealing area, making the process of organizing less of a chore and more of a creative project.

If this appeals to you, let's think about creating a color-coded organizational system that works for you. First of all, decide what categories you need to organize. In an office environment, you might categorize items by project, urgency or type of task, and create color-coded files for each project or task. For the household, you can create a family planner, with categories based on the type of activity, appointment, important event and tasks that need doing, and each member of the family can be assigned a different color.

Creating a color-coded family planner is a great way to involve the whole family in an organization system. It gives each member of the family an easy way to check what they have to do on a daily basis, freeing you from bearing the responsibility of remembering everything for everyone all the time. This should take a weight off your shoulders straight away.

Firstly, decide whether you want a physical chart like a whiteboard or printed calendar, or a digital one like a shared Google Calendar or a spreadsheet. Both have their advantages – the physical planner is always visible, while digital ones can be accessed anywhere and easily kept up-to-date.

Now it's time to assign colors to different tasks and activities, and assign a color to each member of the family. For example:

Parent 1: Light Blue

Parent 2: Dark Green

Child 1: Yellow

Child 2: Purple

Household chores, gardening and grocery shopping: Orange

Homework and work projects: Light Green

Important family events and dates: Red

Health-related dates, e.g. doctors' appointments: Pink

School-related events and dates: Dark Blue

For a weekly chart, you can have columns for each day of the week and rows for each family member, then write in the events, tasks and dates in different colored markers for each day and each person. For a monthly chart you can use a calendar format. Include a legend at the bottom so that everyone knows which color pertains to what, and keep it regularly updated.

If you are using colored sticky labels, you can create a 'completed' section, and move the labels there when they are done. By creating and maintaining a color-coded chart, you and your family can easily visualize and manage the week's schedule, ensuring that all tasks, appointments and events are accounted for and organized effectively.

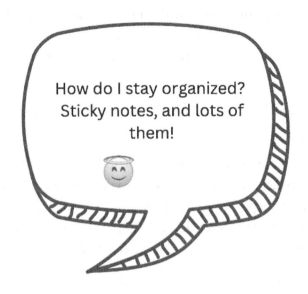

Other Visual Aids

In addition to the planner, visual reminders such as sticky notes or a whiteboard to scribble down reminders are like friendly taps on the shoulder; they're there to catch your eye and gently nudge you towards completing a task. Sticky notes on your bathroom mirror reminding you of your appointments, a weekly meal planner on your fridge door or even a vision board above your desk show-casing your goals can act as both decoration and functional reminders. The key here is to place these reminders in spots you frequently look at. This method harnesses the natural tendency of the ADHD mind to be attracted to visually stimulating items, making sure that your reminders are hard to ignore.

Your environment is another crucial factor in your ability to orga-nize and focus. For visual thinkers, a stimulating and well-orga-nized space can significantly boost productivity. Consider using open shelving in your workspace for color-coded files or bins. Opt for transparent containers in the kitchen for easy visibility. The more visually appealing your environment, the more comfortable and focused you're likely to feel while working in it.

Organizational Tools for Detail-Oriented Individuals

If you are more detail-oriented, using the right tools can make all the difference. Digital tools like Asana and Monday.com allow you to break projects into subtasks and track progress with satisfying precision. These platforms offer the ability to add due dates, assign tasks to team members (or just yourself), and even celebrate with a virtual confetti toss when you complete a task.

But let's not forget about the more old-school tools. A well-structured physical planner can be a haven for the detail-oriented mind. Opt for planners with room for daily, weekly, and monthly overviews so you can make detailed notes and checklists and find them easily when you need them.

Planning is an art form for the detail-oriented individual. It's about foreseeing and arranging the path to your goals. Start with a yearly overview where you jot down key dates and deadlines. From there, zoom in to a monthly breakdown with more specific tasks. Weekly planning sessions allow you to allocate tasks to each day, ensuring every little detail is accounted for. For an added layer of detail, use time blocking within your daily plan to dedicate specific hours to specific tasks—this is especially useful if you're prone to distractions. The trick is to be thorough but flexible; life is unpredictable, and your plan should be a guide, not a prison.

Adapting Strategies for Inattentive ADHD

Perhaps the most effective strategy for those with inattentive ADHD is the use of thematic focus blocks. Instead of a traditional to-do list, you group your activities by theme or type of task and allocate a block of time for each one. For instance, allocate specific hours of the day for work, another block of time solely for creative output, followed by a block for administrative tasks and so on. This can help someone with inattentive ADHD by reducing the number of decisions about what to do next, thus lowering the cognitive load and making it easier to begin a task.

How to create a thematic block-style planner:

1. Start by identifying the major themes you want to work on, such as household chores, work projects, self-care, admin, and so on. Try to group the tasks that naturally go together into one block to simplify decision-making.
2. Next, create a simple schedule with thematic time blocks – typically 'morning', 'early afternoon', 'late afternoon' and 'evening' work well, but you can create your own system.
3. Then, define what needs to be achieved in each block. For example, you could allocate mornings to work-related tasks, spend early afternoons on household management and errands, block out some time for personal projects or hobbies in the late afternoon, and give yourself time in the evening for relaxation and self-care.
4. Some tasks may only need one block per week; others will need to be fitted in every day.
5. Setting specific goals for each block (e.g. finish writing my work report, spending 30 minutes walking in nature) will help to direct your focus and provide a sense of accomplishment when the tasks are completed.

NAME:

DATE:

Weekly Time Block Planner

MORNING 06:00-12:00	M	T	W	T	F	S	S
Morning Routine							
Kids to school/go to work							
Projects and admin							

Afternoon 12:00- 5:00	M	T	W	T	F	S	S
grocery shopping							
hobbies/reading/exercise							

Evening 5:00-10:00	M	T	W	T	F	S	S
dinner & time with family							
evening routine							

This method reduces the cognitive overload that comes from task-switching, allowing your brain to settle comfortably into a focused state. It's also a flexible system, allowing you to shift a task to the next available slot if it takes longer than expected.

While you are working, tools like noise-canceling headphones or focused music playlists can be invaluable. They help create a bubble of concentration, shielding you from the ambient chaos that can easily pull your attention away.

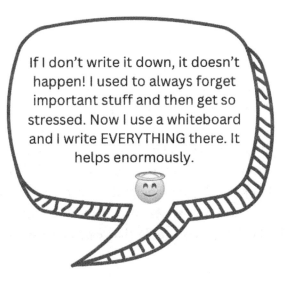

Also, consider using tools that require physical interaction, like whiteboards for brainstorming or paper planners for scheduling. These tools satisfy the need for movement and can make the process of organizing more engaging.

CHAPTER 4

USEFUL TOOLS AND APPS FOR ORGANIZATION

I n the age of smartphones and digital technology, it's as if we have a miniature personal assistant in our pockets, so why not use it to our advantage? There's a plethora of apps and tools designed to bring a semblance of order to our daily lives, and these digital assistants can be very helpful, transforming the daunting mountain of tasks into a series of manageable hills. Let's look at some of the best apps and tools that can make organizing a bit easier.

Note-Taking Apps

For making notes and jotting down ideas, apps like Evernote and Microsoft OneNote can be very helpful. For instance, you can use Evernote to take quick notes during a meeting, and later organize them into different categories for easy reference. Similarly, Microsoft OneNote can be used to create a to-do list for the day, which you can then check off as you complete each task. These apps allow you to capture, organize, and find your notes and ideas across all devices, which is perfect for when your thoughts are racing and your brain's buzzing. These apps often feature organizational tags, voice-to-text options, and even the ability to attach images and links, making them versatile tools in your organizational arsenal.

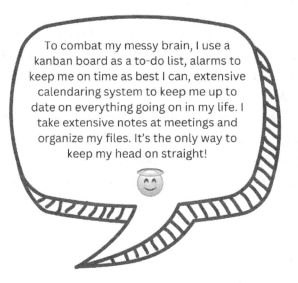

Project Management Apps

Trello and KanbanFlow are project management tools that use boards, lists, and cards to organize and prioritize your projects in a fun, flexible, and rewarding way. These tools are based on the 'Kanban' method, a visual system for managing different jobs as you move through a process. Kanban is a Japanese word that roughly translates as 'card you can see'. You can arrange tasks onto different colored cards and move them around the screen. This can mimic the feeling of moving physical cards around, which can be satisfying and clear for visual thinkers. Customize these apps with colors, labels, and images to make them more personal and visually engaging. These tools help keep your tasks and projects organized and turn the process into a visually interactive experience. It's like turning your to-do list into a visual Pinterest board of productivity, which can be very motivating, especially when you drag a task into the 'Completed' column!

Time Management Apps

Time management apps like Todoist, Goblin Tools and Asana can help to combat the problem of time blindness. These tools allow you to break tasks into subtasks, set priorities, and assign due dates. Todoist, for example, lets you see your tasks in daily or weekly views, which can help visualize how your week is shaping up and where you might need to allocate more focus. What's great about these apps is their reminder systems. You can set multiple alarms for different stages of your task, helping keep time blindness at bay.

List-Making Apps

For those of us who might forget what we were doing two minutes ago, note-taking and list-making apps are our knights in shining armour. Apps like Google Keep or Microsoft To-Do can be fantastic for jotting down everything from sudden bursts of ideas to what you need from the store. Google Keep is particularly handy with its color-coded notes and location-based reminders (imagine your grocery list popping up on your phone the moment you step into the supermarket—magic!). These apps usually offer desktop and smartphone versions that sync seamlessly, ensuring you have your notes no matter which device you're on.

Cleaning and Household Management Apps

There are several innovative apps out there to help streamline cleaning and household management tasks, making them easier and more efficient. Finch combines habit-tracking and goal-setting features to help you establish and maintain a regular cleaning routine. You are given a super-cute virtual pet bird, and for every task you complete your bird gets a reward, which can be very motivating. Sweepy stands out with its user-friendly interface and gamification features, enabling you to assign chores to different members of the household, keep track of what tasks still need to be done, and turn cleaning and decluttering into a game that everyone can participate in. Tody on the other hand, with its traffic light system, excels in visual task management, providing a detailed overview of cleaning tasks and their frequency, helping you to prioritize and tackle tasks before they become over-whelming.

Customization Options

One of the most useful things about these tools is their ability to be customized. Tailoring an app to fit your specific needs can be the difference between it being another unused icon on your screen, or a crucial part of your daily routine. What works for one person might not work for another. You might prefer a minimalistic interface with only the essentials visible, or you might enjoy having all the bells and whistles at your fingertips. The key is to make the app work for you, not the other way around. Take the time to explore the settings in these apps; adjust the notifications, change the themes, or reorganize the layout to suit how you work best. Play around with the settings until you feel the app is truly yours. This might mean turning off certain notifications you find distracting, or setting up custom filters to make your task list less overwhelming. By customizing these tools, you're setting up a digital environment that complements your brain's unique way of processing information, making you more likely to stick with it and become more organized.

I have notes on my Google calendar for appointments, notes on the note section of my phone & alarms I make on my phone for setting trash out, taking my meds, and having to call certain places. Everything I do, I note it someplace that I check several times a day.

Ultimately, these digital tools are not here to add to the chaos, but to simplify our lives. By integrating one or two of these apps and tools into your daily routine, you're equipping yourself with a powerful arsenal against the chaos of ADHD. Whether it's managing your time, keeping track of your tasks, or just remembering to buy milk, there's an app that can help you keep your life running more smoothly. At the end of this chapter, you will find a list of the apps mentioned here, together with others that you might like to explore.

Using a Planner

If you've tried and failed to use a planner because you start with good intentions and end up feeling guilty for not keeping the planner perfectly filled and completed each day, don't despair. One online resource worth checking out is Future ADHD Planning - https://futureadhd.com. Here, you will find a wide range of digital and printable planners specifically created for the ADHD brain and recommended by psychologists, to help you organize in a flexible way that suits you. It has different templates for specific tasks and a daily, weekly and monthly calendar.

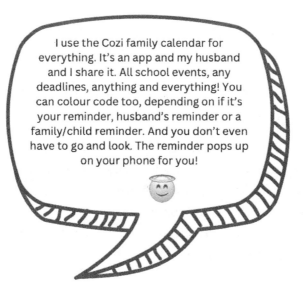

I use the Cozi family calendar for everything. It's an app and my husband and I share it. All school events, any deadlines, anything and everything! You can colour code too, depending on if it's your reminder, husband's reminder or a family/child reminder. And you don't even have to go and look. The reminder pops up on your phone for you!

Another planner app that works well is Cozi (https://www.cozi.com), designed as a family organizer that helps manage various aspects of family life in a way everyone can use. You start by creating an account that all family members can access. Each member can log in using their email address. One of the main features of Cozi is its shared calendar. Family members can add, view, and manage events that are visible to everyone, such as important school events, doctor's appointments, extracurricular activities, and so on. You can also create multiple to-do lists, shopping lists and meal planners that everyone can access, share and contribute to. The journal feature is another nice touch – anyone can create a shared journal entry to record a family moment, with photos and descriptions. You can also set reminders and notifications so that nobody misses an important appointment. Finally, each family member can be assigned a specific color, making it easier to see at a glance who's doing what.

Reviewing and Reminding

Once a week, it's worth taking 5 or 10 minutes to review all the coming week's commitments in your planner. This will not only remind you of the must-dos, the fixed appointments and important meetings, but it can also be a real eye-opener, helping you see how much you're trying to pack into your days.

With ADHD, it's easy to overestimate what you can handle in a day or a week, leading to a packed schedule that leaves little room for downtime or unexpected tasks. By using a planner, then stepping back and assessing your commitments, you can start to find balance, ensuring you have time for both work and play without stretching yourself too thin.

Here's a list of some of the best digital apps and tools out there to help with organization:

Great for visual organizers:

1. Trello – https://www.trello.com

- Trello is a versatile project management tool that organizes tasks and projects using boards, lists, and cards. It's very visual, which can help track priorities and progress.
- **How it works**: You can create boards for different projects or areas of your life, add lists to each board for tasks or stages of a project, and then add cards for each task. Cards can be moved between lists as they progress.

2. KanbanFlow – https://kanbanflow.com

- KanbanFlow is a project management app that uses the Kanban methodology. It allows you to visualize your workflow, track tasks, and manage projects using Kanban boards.
- **How it works**: Kanban is a visual system of colored cards that allows you to keep track of your work as you move through a job or project.

3. Monday.com – https://www.monday.com

- Monday.com is a popular work management platform that helps individuals and teams plan, track, and collaborate on projects and tasks.
- **How it works**: Using a visual board layout with various views (Kanban, Gantt, calendar, etc.), teams can customize

their workflows, automate processes, and integrate with other tools.

4. MindMeister – www.mindmeister.com

- MindMeister is a mind-mapping app that lets you capture, organize and share ideas visually.
- **How it works**: You can create diagrams that represent ideas, tasks or projects, either from scratch or from templates, and import existing files to integrate into the mind map.

Great for list-making and organizing tasks:

5. Evernote – https://evernote.com

- Evernote is a note-taking app that helps you organize your personal and professional projects. It allows you to store notes, documents, photos, and web pages in one place.
- **How it works**: You can create notebooks for various topics and add notes to them. Notes can include text, images, audio, and attachments. They're also searchable, making it easy to find what you need.

6. Notion – https://www.notion.so

- Notion combines note-taking, task management, databases and spreadsheets to create a flexible and comprehensive organizational tool.
- **How it works**: You can create pages and databases to manage different aspects of your life or work. Each page can be customized with different blocks for tasks, notes, calendars and more.

7. Microsoft OneNote – https://www.onenote.com

- OneNote works like a digital notebook that gathers users' notes, drawings, screen clips and audio commentaries and makes them searchable.
- **How it works**: OneNote allows you to create multiple notebooks, each with its own sections and pages, much like a physical notebook. You can type or handwrite notes, insert images, audio and video and use drawing tools.

8.. Microsoft To-Do – https://to-do.office.com

- Microsoft To-Do is a task management app that helps you manage, prioritize and complete tasks. You can create to-do lists, set reminders, and track deadlines.
- **How it works**: To-Do allows you to create different lists to organize tasks based on categories, projects or contexts. Within each list, you can add subtasks, set due dates and add notes or attachments.

9. Google Keep – https://keep.google.com

- Google Keep is a straightforward note-taking and task-management app that is great for quick notes and to-do lists. It can be accessed from any device.
- **How it works**: You can create notes and lists, add images and audio and set reminders.

Great for Time Management:

10. Asana – https://asana.com

- Asana is more focused on the work environment. It helps manage tasks and projects across teams, making it great for professional use. It contains task lists, timelines, calendars and more.
- **How it works**: You can create projects, add tasks, assign due dates, and set reminders. It also allows for collaboration with others.

11. Todoist – https://todoist.com

- Todoist is a task manager that's built around simplicity and flexibility. It allows you to manage tasks and projects anywhere, on any device.
- **How it works**: You can create tasks, organize them into projects, set priority levels and due dates, and integrate with other apps.

12. Goblin Tools – https://goblin.tools

- Goblin Tools has been specially designed for neurodivergent users. It breaks the to-do list down into smaller, more manageable steps to simplify day-to-day tasks.
- **How it works**: Each task has a 'spiciness level' from 1 to 5, depending on how much breaking down it needs. In addition, there are features such as 'the Compiler', which helps to formalize thoughts into actionable tasks, and 'the Chef', which can create recipes based on the ingredients you have available at the time.

Good for Planning, Tracking Habits and Maintaining Focus:

13. Forest App – https://www.forestapp.cc

- Forest App is designed to help you stay focused and present. It's beneficial for those who are easily distracted.
- **How it works**: The app allows you to set a timer for however long you want to focus, and as you work, you grow a virtual tree. If you leave the app to check your phone, the tree dies. It's a great motivational tool for sticking to a task.

14. Future ADHD Planner - https://futureadhd.com

- Future ADHD Planner provides a range of digital and downloadable planners specifically tailored to the ADHD brain.
- **How it works**: You can opt for a digital planner that works with your iPad or phone, or download a physical paper planner. Either way, there are lots of different options to choose from.

15. Cozi – https://www.cozi.com

- Cozi bills itself as the #1 organizing app for families.
- **How it works**: With a shared family calendar and features such as communal to-do lists, shopping lists, meal planners and recipes, a family journal, and color-coding, this is a great way for families to stay coordinated in one user-friendly space.

Good for Cleaning and Keeping Track of Household Tasks:

16. Sweepy – https://sweepy.app

- Sweepy is a home cleaning schedule app designed to help manage and organize household tasks.
- **How it works**: Sweepy allows you to create a customizable cleaning schedule, split chores among family members and even turn the routine into a game to make it more fun – you earn virtual coins for each task completed, which you can spend on decorating a virtual room. The app tracks the cleanliness of each room, prioritizes tasks and automatically generates a daily schedule to help overcome overwhelm and maintain focus.

17. Finch – https://finchcare.com

- Finch is a self-care app that encourages you to take care of yourself by taking care of a super-cute pet bird. It acts a self-care journal and task motivator with lots of different fun prompts to encourage you to set goals and complete tasks.
- **How it works**: If you are feeling low or unmotivated and have a particular task you want to complete, you can set it as a goal on Finch. When you've completed the job, your pet bird gets a reward – food, little outfits and so on.

18. Tody – https://todyapp.com

- Tody is an app that turns cleaning into a game. It visualizes dirtiness to motivate cleaning, and visualizes the effect of cleaning to give you satisfaction when you have completed your tasks.

- **How it works**: The app has a traffic light system of 'red', 'amber' and 'green' that it assigns to different tasks, so that you can prioritize which ones to start first. It tracks your chores and gives suggestions and reminders.

19. Dubbii – https://www.dubii.app

- Dubbii is a body doubling app with step-by-step body doubling videos for tasks like decluttering and cleaning, to help you get started and stay on track.
- **How it works**: The app asks you 'what do you need help with today?' You choose from a range of videos such as 'laundry', 'making the bed' etc., and the video walks you through the task, breaking down each stage into micro-actions, and acting as a virtual body double to help you keep going. When you have completed a task, you earn badges.

20. The Organized Mum – https://theorganizedmum.com

- The Organized Mum is based around an app, The Organized Mum Rocks (TOM), which is billed as a 'personal trainer for your housework'.
- **How it works**: There are lots of different guided cleans and audio sessions to choose from for cooking, cleaning and organizing. The app features prompts, playlists and customizable task lists, and you can track your progress and earn rewards as you go.

CHAPTER 5

KICK-STARTING YOUR ORGANIZATIONAL JOURNEY: THE MORNING ROUTINE

I magine it's one of those mornings where even your coffee needs a coffee. Your alarm clock is buzzing, the bed is cosy, and the day's to-do list looms like a mountain. But what if, instead of letting the chaos dictate your day, you had a simple and easy-to-follow morning routine that you didn't have to think about too much, to help you get the day off to a positive start? This chapter is about turning those groggy mornings into a launchpad for success with a dash of intentionality and a sprinkle of ADHD adaptability.

The Simple and Easy Morning Routine

Creating a good morning routine that works for you sets a positive tone for the day ahead. Here are some suggestions for a basic, balanced morning routine that you can adapt according to your personal preferences and schedule. Please note - you don't have to do it all! This is a list of options – you can choose the ones that you feel are achievable on a regular basis and that speak to you.

1. **Set the alarm and try to wake up early**. Waking up around the same time every day, even on weekends, helps to regulate your body clock and can improve your overall sleep quality.

2. **Hydrate**. Start your day with a glass of water. Overnight, your body, especially your brain, gets dehydrated, so it's beneficial to keep a glass of water by your bed and drink it first thing in the morning.

3. **Engage in some form of physical activity for a few minutes**. Gentle stretching exercises, a short morning walk, or a brief yoga session will invigorate both your body and your mind.

4. **Meditate**. Spend a few minutes meditating, practising deep breathing or doing a mindfulness exercise to clear your mind, reduce stress and prepare for the day.

5. **Eat a healthy breakfast**. Fuel your body with a nutritious breakfast with a good balance of proteins, fats and carbohydrates. A protein-rich breakfast is particularly beneficial to people with ADHD.

6. **Personal Care**. Follow a simple, quick grooming routine: shower, brush your teeth, do your hair, and get dressed. This helps you feel fresh and signals to your brain that it's time to start the day.

7. **Avoid screens in the first hour**. Try to avoid jumping straight into emails, news or social media. Giving yourself a screen-free first hour can reduce early morning stress and distraction.

8. **Plan your day**. Take a few minutes to review your tasks and priorities. This can help you manage your time effectively and feel more prepared and focused.

Simple Morning Routine

- [ ] Wake up early.

- [ ] Drink a glass of water.

- [ ] Stretch and do some light exercise.

- [ ] Make your bed.

- [ ] Eat a nutritious breakfast.

- [ ] Take a shower and get dressed.

- [ ] Avoid screens in the first hour.

- [ ] Set goals and plan your day.

The 5-minute Morning Mental Prep – Planning the Day Ahead

Taking 5 minutes in the morning to plan your day and set your intentions can make all the difference to how the day goes. You might be wondering, "what's the big deal about setting intentions?" Well, think of them as your personal road signs for the day ahead —they help guide your actions and mindset. For those who are juggling the dynamic duo of everyday life and ADHD, setting intentions can be really helpful. It's like programming your internal GPS each morning to navigate the day's challenges more effectively. By starting your day with clear intentions, you're more likely to stay aligned with your goals and less likely to be derailed by distractions or overwhelm.

Start by finding a quiet spot, like a corner of your bedroom. Sit down with a notebook or your favorite digital device and jot down two or three intentions for the day. These could be as simple as, "Today, I will clear the kitchen surfaces and sort through the mail on the kitchen table," or they could be more emotional: "I will be kinder to myself today." The key is to keep the tasks achievable and the intentions tied to what you need to focus on the most.

Next, think about priorities for the day ahead. When everything feels urgent, nothing is. Try the "Must, Should, Could" method to cut through the noise. Write down all the tasks you need to do. Then, categorize them into 'Must do', 'Should do', and 'Could do'. 'Must do' tasks have immediate deadlines or significant conse-quences if delayed (like unmissable appointments or finishing a work project). 'Should do' tasks are important but can wait if necessary (like organizing your workspace), and 'Could do' tasks would be nice to get done but aren't urgent (like sorting through old emails). This method helps to break down your tasks and see where to focus your energy first. It's a simple, visual way to plan your day, giving your brain a clear path to follow.

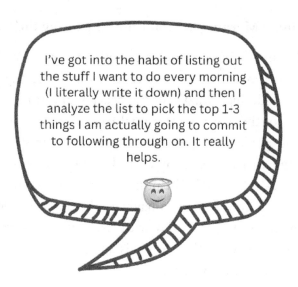

Visualization Techniques

To amplify the power of your intentions, pair them with visualization. This technique isn't just for athletes or performers; it's a potent tool for anyone, especially those with ADHD who might struggle with focus and motivation. Visualizing how you want your day to unfold can cement your intentions in your mind. Close your eyes and imagine yourself successfully navigating the day's tasks. See yourself moving seamlessly from one activity to another, handling disruptions with grace, and ending the day feeling accomplished. This mental rehearsal primes your brain to act in ways that align with your visualized outcomes, making it easier to manage ADHD symptoms throughout the day.

Adjusting Intentions Based on Needs

One of the superpowers of having ADHD is being highly attuned to how different days bring different energy levels and challenges. That's why it's crucial to tailor your daily intentions based on your current mental and physical state. Some days, your intention might be about productivity, while other days, it might be about self-care or simply trying to be present. Check in with yourself each morning—how do you feel, what's on your plate for the day, and what challenges might arise? Adjust your intentions accordingly. If you didn't get enough sleep, maybe set an intention to take breaks, or to approach work in shorter segments or better still, give yourself permission to take a power nap. By aligning your intentions with your state of being, you create a flexible framework that supports you in managing your ADHD effectively throughout the day.

These morning minutes are your opportunity to steer the day in your favor right from the start. By setting intentions, you're not just planning your actions; you're also aligning your mindset with your goals, which is especially powerful for managing ADHD. This simple practice can transform your day from reactive to proactive, giving you a sense of control and accomplishment. So, before the world rushes in tomorrow morning, take those five minutes. Set your intentions, visualize your success, and watch your day unfold with more purpose and less chaos.

CHAPTER 6

THE POWER OF 5 MINUTES: STARTING SMALL FOR BIG WINS

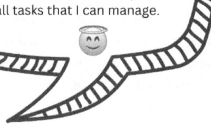

When I have larger chunks of time I keep going for longer, because my 5-minute tasks make it easier. There are times when I can only do 15 minutes, but other times I can get a lot done, because I break it up into small tasks that I can manage.

S o now let's dive into the real game-changer: the power of five minutes. Yes, just five minutes! It sounds almost too good to be true, but the magic in managing ADHD isn't in overhauling your entire life in one fell swoop; it's in the beauty of small, achievable goals.

When you're staring down a task that seems as daunting as climbing Mount Everest in flip-flops, knowing where to start is half the battle. It's easy to feel overwhelmed or unmotivated, especially when your ADHD brain is pulling you in a million different directions. The trick to overcoming that initial resistance is to simplify the task to such an extent that beginning doesn't seem so formidable. This approach reduces the pressure and the mental load, making it easier to begin—and often, once you've started, continuing doesn't seem so tough.

You *can* make a significant dent in your organizational goals in just five minutes. It's not about completing the entire task; it's about breaking the inertia of inactivity and starting with small, manageable steps.

Small steps are your secret weapon. They transform the monstrous task of organizing a year's worth of paperwork into sorting just a few papers today, a few tomorrow, and then, before you know it, you're done. This method is not only more manageable but also less daunting. It builds confidence piece by piece—or paper by paper. Consider this: if you decided to organize just one drawer in your dresser, that's a task that can be done in around 5 minutes, and once you see that neat drawer, you'll feel a boost of accomplishment. That's your small win and your hit of dopamine.

In five minutes, you could clear a small section of your desk, sort through your mail, or decide which of your pens still work and which should meet the trash can. These are all quick tasks, but once you start and finish them, the sense of achievement is dispro-portionately satisfying compared to the time invested.

This is about tricking your brain into getting started, which is often the most challenging part. The principle is simple: it's easier to commit to a five-minute task than to an hour-long marathon. Once you start, you often find the momentum to keep going, or at the very least, you'll have made a dent.

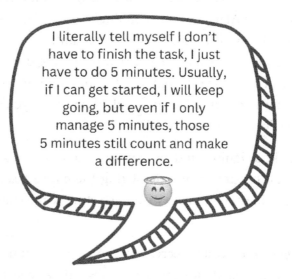

Rewarding Success – the Power of the Dopamine Hit

Celebrating each success plays a crucial role in this approach. Giving yourself a small treat or a break after completing each task is all part of the process. This positive reinforcement releases a hit of dopamine that makes the brain light up like a Christmas tree. It's about creating a positive association with the tasks you've accomplished. This is vital because it transforms your perspective on organizing from a dreaded chore to an activity that brings tangible rewards.

These rewards don't have to be big; they just need to be meaningful to you. It could be something as simple as a cup of tea and some downtime to read a magazine or a chapter of a book, time set aside for crafting, or going outside for a walk in the fresh air. For bigger tasks you could treat yourself to a night out. You could even assign a small amount of money to certain tasks, and when you have completed them, you can spend the money you have earned on something you really want, just for yourself. These rewards are crucial - they act as a little pat on the back from yourself to yourself, acknowledging your efforts and encouraging you to keep pushing forward.

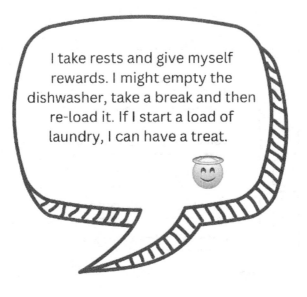

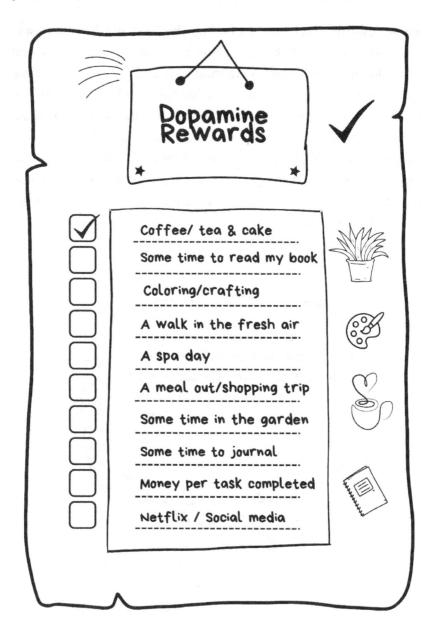

Dopamine Rewards

- [x] Coffee/ tea & cake
- [ ] Some time to read my book
- [ ] Coloring/crafting
- [ ] A walk in the fresh air
- [ ] A spa day
- [ ] A meal out/shopping trip
- [ ] Some time in the garden
- [ ] Some time to journal
- [ ] Money per task completed
- [ ] Netflix / Social media

Furthermore, each little success builds momentum, turning the tide in your favor. As these victories accumulate, they start to form a new habit, a new way of life that gradually leads to more considerable successes. Think of it as your personal success snowball. Each victory adds size and speed to the snowball, making it easier to tackle larger tasks down the line. For instance, once you've managed to keep that one drawer organized, you'll find yourself motivated to tackle the closet. And after the closet, who knows? Maybe you'll move on to the garage or the attic. It's about building up your organizational muscle, one small lift at a time, until before you know it, you're lifting heavier weights with ease.

It's helpful to track your progress in a notebook or digital diary to make these victories genuinely impactful. This isn't just about crossing tasks off a list – although that in itself can be very satisfying – it's about visually and tangibly seeing how your efforts add up over time, which can be incredibly motivating. One effective way to do this is by maintaining a success journal. At the end of each day, jot down the organizational tasks you've completed. This could be anything from clearing out the kitchen cupboard to setting up a new way to keep track of your appointments. Over time, flipping through this journal can give you a concrete sense of how far you've come, turning the intangible into something you can see and touch.

Another effective method is to create a visual progress board. This can be a physical board in your workspace or a digital one on your computer or phone. Each task or project gets a card or a note, and you move these from one side of the board to the other as you progress. Watching your tasks physically move from 'To-Do' to 'Done' provides a clear visual representation of your progress and can be a real boost to your morale. And it all starts with just five minutes.

CHAPTER 7

OVERCOMING TASK PARALYSIS AND PROCRASTINATION: THE POWER OF THE 5-MINUTE TASK

You know, I used to really struggle with keeping on top of things around the house. The clutter and mess just felt so overwhelming, I didn't even know where to start.
But then I had this realization - I didn't have to do it all at once! That's when I decided to take baby steps instead...

...So here's what I started doing: every day, I'd do something for 5 minutes, take a break and do another 5 minutes, three times in total. So I spend just 15 minutes per day doing a quick clean-up. Nothing crazy, just straightening up a bit. Then I'd make sure to run a load of dishes and a load of laundry. And I committed to getting rid of 10 things per day, either donating them or trashing them...

...Honestly, at first I thought "this isn't going to make a difference. But it really started adding up. Before I knew it, I could actually open the door without that pit of dread in my stomach.
In the past, I avoided even trying because I couldn't tackle it all immediately. But doing a little bit consistently? It changes everything...

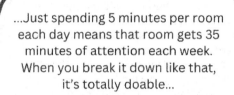

...Just spending 5 minutes per room each day means that room gets 35 minutes of attention each week. When you break it down like that, it's totally doable...

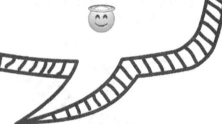

...I'm not going to lie, some days I really don't feel like it.
But I stick with my little routine and it's paying off big time.
Now my house feels manageable instead of like this huge overwhelming beast.

P icture this: you're standing in front of what I affectionately call 'Mount Laundry'—that ever-growing pile of clothes that seems to have a life of its own. The sheer size of it could easily make you want to turn around, crawl back into bed, and forget you ever thought of tackling laundry today. This is what many people with ADHD know all too well as task paralysis. It's that all-consuming dread that washes over you when you think about starting a task that feels too big, too overwhelming, or too complex.

Understanding task paralysis in ADHD is like peeling back the layers of a complex puzzle. It's not about laziness or a lack of motivation, as some might wrongly assume. It's often about how our brains perceive and process tasks. When a task appears enormous or vague, the ADHD brain can freeze, unsure where to start or fearful of not completing it perfectly. This response is a protective mechanism, almost like the brain's way of saying, "this feels risky; let's avoid it altogether." But, as we know, avoidance only leads to more stress and less getting done. The relief comes when we realize that this is not a personal failing, but a common challenge for many with ADHD. This understanding can lift a huge weight off your shoulders, allowing you to approach the problem with a mindset geared towards solutions rather than self-blame.

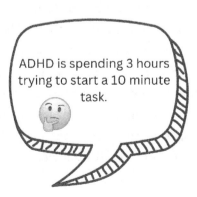

ADHD is spending 3 hours trying to start a 10 minute task.

So, how do we combat this paralysis? The trick lies in breaking down the monstrous blob of a task into smaller, bite-sized pieces that have a clear beginning and an end. I'm talking about 5-minute micro-tasks that feel so doable that you'd think, "Why not just do it?" For instance, instead of facing the whole mountain of laundry, commit to sorting just the socks. Yes, just the socks. This micro-task reduces the cognitive load, making it easier to start and less likely to trigger overwhelm. And once you start and finish this tiny task, you've scored a quick win against task paralysis. This win creates a ripple effect, often motivating you to tackle the next small task, maybe the t-shirts next, folding the towels, and so on. The sense of accomplishment that comes from these small victories can be a powerful motivator, encouraging you to keep going.

Before embarking on any task, take a moment to visualize yourself completing it. This mental rehearsal primes your brain for action, reducing the anxiety and overwhelm often associated with the task. Visualization not only prepares you mentally but also adjusts your emotional state, making you more resilient against the paralysis that often hits before a task.

Tackling Procrastination: 5-Minute Strategies to Begin Any Task.

Procrastination isn't about laziness or poor time management; for the ADHD brain, it's often a more complex beast. Faced with a task that seems too mundane or too colossal, a person with ADHD will experience a spike in anxiety, leading to avoidance behavior. The dopamine-driven circuits in our brain crave instant gratification, and let's be honest, most organizational tasks don't deliver immediate, thrilling rewards. This can make starting such tasks seem even less appealing, creating a vicious cycle of delay and disappointment.

So, how do we break this cycle? It begins with acknowledging that procrastination isn't a personal failing but a common challenge for many with ADHD. One effective strategy we have already looked at is spending a few minutes each morning writing down a set of clear, achievable goals for each day. This clarity reduces the mental clutter that can paralyze your start. It's important to approach this process with self-compassion. Be kind to yourself and understand that overcoming procrastination is a journey, not a one-time fix.

Conquering Procrastination: The Power of the Five-Minute Commitment

The key to breaking the cycle of procrastination is to make starting as easy as possible. This is where the magic of the five-minute commitment comes into play. Set a timer and promise yourself that you'll tackle the task for just five minutes. Often, the hardest part is just getting started; once you're in motion, it's easier to keep going. This method helps build momentum, and before you know it, you might find yourself wanting to continue beyond the initial five minutes.

Timers are not just about tracking time; they serve as a psychological trigger, creating a sense of urgency that helps focus your mind. For those who have ADHD, understanding that there's a finite start and end time can make a task feel less daunting. It's like telling your brain, "Hey, it's just five minutes. We can handle that." This bounded time frame helps to alleviate the anxiety of feeling like the task will drag on indefinitely, which can be a significant deterrent to getting started.

Time yourself doing a task (especially the ones you hate/struggle with). I started timing how long it takes me to unload the dishwasher and was able to provide concrete evidence to myself that it actually isn't that bad. It takes me 5 mins or less. I did this for over a month and now that pit in my stomach that accompanies thinking about the dishes is almost non existent.

Altering your environment can also significantly improve your ability to start tasks. A cluttered workspace can be incredibly distracting and demotivating. Take a moment to create a setting that encourages productivity. This might mean clearing your desk of unnecessary items, closing tabs on your computer that you don't need, or even changing your physical location. Sometimes, a change of scenery can be just what you need to refresh your mind and reduce the temptation to procrastinate. If you're struggling to start a task in your home office, try moving to the kitchen table or even a local café. A new environment can provide a new perspective, making the task feel more manageable.

Moreover, consider the sensory aspects of your environment. Music helps many people enormously: with your most upbeat playlist on full blast, any job feels less of a chore.

For some with ADHD, background noise, like a busy coffee shop, paradoxically enhances focus, while for others, a quiet room with minimal distractions works better. Experiment with different settings to find what helps you concentrate best. Organizing your tools and materials before starting can also help. If everything you need is within easy reach, for example a basic set of cleaning products in every room, the task will seem less cumbersome, and you'll be more likely to dive in without hesitation.

Remember to reward yourself whenever you have completed a task. Take a break and do something you love for a few minutes. By routinely breaking tasks down into micro-actions, rewarding yourself for small victories, and using visualization to prep your mind, you transform your approach to daunting tasks. No longer are they insurmountable mountains of dread, but rather a series of small hills, each manageable, each conquerable. This approach doesn't just help you overcome procrastination and task paralysis – it rebuilds your relationship with tasks and productivity, turning what was once overwhelming into something you can confidently manage, one small step at a time.

Continue this process for each area you need to organize, always breaking down larger tasks into smaller, manageable chunks, and always starting with the first five minutes. Remember, the key here is consistency, not speed. It's about making steady progress that you can build on, rather than trying to do everything all at once and burning out. Think of it as laying bricks. Each task you complete is another brick in the structure of your organized life, and every brick counts, no matter how small.

CHAPTER 8

SETTING UP FOR TOMORROW: THE 5-MINUTE EVENING ROUTINE

I magine easing into your evening with a sense of calm, knowing that tomorrow's tasks are neatly arranged and ready for you. That's the power of a well-crafted evening routine, especially for those with ADHD, where a little preparation can significantly reduce tomorrow morning's chaos and decision fatigue. Let's talk about being kind to your future self, and turning those crucial evening minutes into a springboard for a smoother tomorrow.

The Power of Preparation

The secret to a stress-free morning is often in the groundwork laid the night before. Preparing for the next day can shift your mornings from hectic to harmonious, reducing the mental load that often comes with starting the day. This preparation might involve deciding on and setting out tomorrow's outfit, pre-packing lunches, or jotting down a quick to-do list for the next day. Each of these actions diminishes the number of decisions you need to make in the morning, conserving that precious mental energy for more demanding tasks as the day progresses. This streamlined approach can be a game-changer, setting a positive tone for the entire day, especially for those who might struggle with decision-making, or become easily overwhelmed by too many choices.

A Simple Evening Routine

So, what does an effective evening routine look like? It's simple and quick and focuses on key preparations that make a big difference.

1. **Start by doing a quick brain dump**. Spend five or ten minutes writing down everything that's on your mind that you need to remember for the next day – tasks, appointments, reminders and anything else cluttering your brain. We'll look in more detail at the art of the brain dump in chapter 17.
2. **Identify the top three most important tasks or priorities**. Look over what you have just written and mark the three most important items with a star, or highlight them so you won't forget them.
3. **Check the weather for the next day**. This can help you make practical decisions about what to wear and whether you need to allow extra time for your commute.
4. **Make some basic preparations**. If you have an important appointment or meeting you need to prepare for, spend a few minutes thinking about what you'll need to take with you.
5. **Check what the kids need for school the next day**. Make sure their lunchbox, sports gear, and other items are ready for the morning.

6. **Place any essentials—keys, wallet, work materials— near the door**. This acts as your launchpad for the next day, ensuring you can grab and go without a second thought.

These steps are small, but they help automate your morning process, making it more efficient and less prone to forgetfulness or frantic searches that can often start the day on a stressful note. Spending just a few minutes each evening setting these things up will create a buffer against the morning rush, which can be particularly stressful for an ADHD mind.

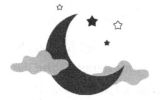

A SIMPLE & EFFECTIVE BEDTIME ROUTINE

1.Start by doing a quick sweep of the kitchen and living room. Spend 5 minutes picking up stuff from the floor and counters. Fill and start the dishwasher.

2. Do a brain dump. Spend five or ten minutes writing down everything that's on your mind that you need to remember for the next day – tasks, appointments, reminders and anything else cluttering your brain.

3. Look over what you have just written and mark the three most important items with a star, or highlight them so you won't forget them tomorrow.

4. Check the weather for the next day. This can help you make practical decisions about what to wear and whether you need to allow extra time for your commute.

5. Make some basic preparations. If you have an important appointment you need to prepare for, spend a few minutes thinking about what you'll need.

6. If you have kids, check what they need for school the next day. Make sure their lunchbox, sports gear, and other items are ready for the morning.

7. Place any essentials—keys, wallet, work materials—near the door. This acts as your launchpad for the next day, ensuring you can grab and go without a second thought.

Reflecting on the Day's Successes and Challenges

Incorporating a brief reflection into your evening routine can also be beneficial. This isn't about dwelling on every detail of the day, but instead taking a moment to acknowledge what went well and what could be improved. Did you find a new way to overcome a distraction? Did a particular task take longer than expected? Recognizing these patterns can provide valuable insights that help you adjust your strategies and expectations, making you more adept at managing your ADHD symptoms over time.

This reflection can be as simple as mentally acknowledging these moments or jotting them down in a journal. The act of writing can be particularly therapeutic, helping to clear your mind and set a positive intention for the next day. It's a chance to celebrate the wins, learn from the challenges, and continually refine your approach to living with ADHD. And then we can follow Ralph Waldo Emerson's advice: "Finish each day and be done with it. You have done what you could. Some blunders and absurdities no doubt crept in, forget them as soon as you can. Tomorrow is a new day."

CHAPTER 9
DECLUTTERING 101 - THE DOOM PILE

W e've all been there. Standing in front of a large pile of clutter, wondering whether your kid's science folder, the phone charger, the missing shoe or the unpaid electricity bill is submerged somewhere in its depths. Welcome to the DOOM pile (Didn't Organize, Only Moved), a seemingly random heap of objects that have accumulated over time. These piles usually consist of items that don't have a designated storage space, or things that you've set aside with the intention of dealing with later but never quite got around to. Papers, books, clothes, gadgets, you name it – the junk together with the super-important – and all randomly mixed together in an unorganized heap. No wonder they are called 'doom piles' because it's often when we have to confront them that our sense of dread and overwhelm goes into overdrive.

The doom pile is a visual reminder of two of the key difficulties of ADHD, the challenge of procrastination and struggles with decision-making and organization. These piles often form in places where you tend to drop things 'just for now'. As the pile grows, so does the overwhelm, and we are reluctant to start tackling the pile because it is too intimidating. The good news is that you are not alone, and there are ways to conquer these piles of chaos.

But before we dive in, let's spend some time getting our decluttering toolkit ready. Having the right tools can make the daunting task of decluttering more manageable and even enjoyable. By having everything you need at hand, you can stay focused and efficient and make steady progress toward a clutter-free environment.

Decluttering

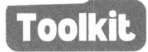

For your Decluttering Toolkit, you will need:

- Four large sorting containers – boxes or bins labelled 'Keep', 'Donate', 'Trash' and a 'Maybe' box for the items you can't decide on immediately. Also, a smaller box to store photos and other important documents.

- Basic cleaning supplies like trash bags, multi-surface cleaner and microfiber cloths, gloves, paper towels and a hand-held vacuum cleaner.

- Storage solutions like empty plastic boxes, bags and open shelves, plus labels and a marker pen.

- A timer and a great playlist, audiobook or podcast.

- Donation bags to transport items to donation centers.

- If you are clearing the home office, you will need sticky notes, files and folders.

Don't forget to have a really good reward in mind for when you have completed your decluttering tasks, to help keep you motivated!

Let's Talk About Wall Hanging Organizers

Hanging organizers with multiple pockets for the kitchen, bathroom, closet and office, either clear plastic or with fabric pockets, can be life-savers.

- On the kitchen cupboard door you can hang a clear plastic set of pockets to store sauces, seasonings, jars and other items that otherwise get lost in the back of the cupboard.
- In the bathroom, your shampoo, hair masks, bubble bath, make-up remover pads, nail polish and so on will be easy to store and quick to find.
- In the hallway, all those small but important items that so often get lost – keys, phone chargers, glasses, can be popped into the pockets and easily found again.
- For the kids' room, these hanging pockets can be used to store smaller toys, gaming remotes and those all-important Lego figurines.

I got some hanging pockets and it's been life changing to have designated spots for things like sunscreen, make-up, medicine etc. I can't believe how much time I save not searching for things, and how much money I save not buying things I already have, but don't know where to find them!

Tips for using your Decluttering Toolkit

1. Keep it accessible – place your storage boxes in an easy-to-reach place so you can throw items into a box whenever you feel the urge.
2. Restock regularly – make sure to replace consumables like trash bags and cleaning supplies as needed.
3. Personalize your kit – adjust and add to the contents based on your specific needs.
4. Duplicate as much as possible so that you have the supplies you need ready and waiting for you in each room.

The Emotional Side of Decluttering

Before we start, a word about our emotional attachment to stuff. Too much of it is an energy sucker and can easily become a source of stress. The truth is that the less stuff you own, the less stuff you have to tidy. That's not to say we all have to become minimalists, but we do sometimes need to be ruthless and clear out the clutter, even though it is often really hard.

I want you to know that you DO HAVE PERMISSION to throw things away. You are not obligated to keep every note, every gift, every photo, every child's drawing. If you throw something out, it doesn't make you a bad person. You are making your space clearer, cleaner and better for yourself and your family, and that's a huge gift. There are some really precious objects that we will keep forever, but most of our stuff is temporary. It has its place and its use in our lives for a certain time, and then it is time to let it go, either to the great garbage pile in the sky, or to another home for a new family to use and enjoy. We need to know that this is ok, and a normal part of life.

So, first up, find the doom pile that feels the most urgent, and then identify a section of that pile that you want to tackle. Put on some music, take a deep breath and pick up your first item. Sometimes, it's easy – the empty pizza boxes and out-of-date magazines are an instant 'throw'. Other items are harder to place, and you might find yourself getting stuck at some point, not knowing what to do with a particular item that seems too good to throw out but not good enough to keep. For these items, here are 10 Key Questions you can ask when deciding whether to keep it or throw it out. Try to answer as honestly as you can.

The Essential Decluttering Questions:

1. Have I used it in the last year?
2. Do I need this to be productive or happy?
3. Is it less than $30, and would it take less than 30 minutes to replace (on Amazon, at WalMart, etc)?
4. If I lost it, would I buy it again?
5. Do I have other items that do the same thing?
6. Do I have space for it?
7. Do I have it "just to have it"?
8. Would someone else benefit from it more than me?
9. What is the real reason I am keeping it?
10. Is it worth the effort of dusting?

These questions help you evaluate each possession mindfully. Asking, 'do I use or love this item?' gets to the heart of whether you should keep it or not. We could sum this up by saying 'if you don't love it or use it, it's clutter'. The goal is to identify what no longer serves its purpose, to create a clearer, happier, and more clutter-free space without guilt. As a wise person once said, your home is a living space, not a storage facility.

Two Tried-and-Tested Decluttering Methods

There are two decluttering gurus out there who have perfected systems of tidying and organizing that have helped countless people deal with the problem of too much stuff. You've probably heard of them, and maybe you've even bought their books. For those of you who haven't read the books, I've created a summary of both systems and extracted the most useful advice, so that you can easily incorporate it into your own decluttering plan.

Firstly, let's look at Dana K. White, whose books *Decluttering at the Speed of Life* and *How to Manage Your Home Without Losing Your Mind* have sold hundreds of thousands of copies. She has developed a practical, realistic approach to decluttering that resonates especially well with those who struggle with traditional organizing methods.

At the heart of the method is the Container Concept. She teaches that the purpose of a container – a drawer, a shelf, a storage box, even a whole room – is to set limits on the amount of stuff you keep. For example, if you have a bookshelf, the bookshelf is the container. Only keep as many books as will neatly fit on the shelf. If there are more books than bookshelves, you need to decide which books are most valuable or useful to you and let go of the rest. There are three main stages to this method:

1. Define the container – identify the space or container where a group of items will be stored.
2. Set limits – only keep what comfortably fits inside that container. If it doesn't fit, it needs to go.
3. Prioritize – Keep the most important and useful items first. Anything that doesn't fit after that should be considered for donation or disposal.

There are several specific steps in this method to clear clutter efficiently.

Do the easy stuff first. Starting with easy items reduces overwhelm and builds momentum. Begin with items that are obvious trash or belong somewhere else. Quickly removing these items creates visible progress.

- **For example**: Pick up that pile of old magazines and put them in the recycle bin, throw away the empty soda cans, and hang up the coat in the middle of the floor.

Make a 'Donate' Box and keep it easily accessible as you come across items you no longer need or use.

- **For example**: old clothes, duplicate kitchen gadgets, toys your children no longer play with – put them directly in the Donate box and take the box regularly to your local donation center.

Identify areas where clutter tends to accumulate due to procrastination. Focus on one area at a time where things pile up because you put off dealing with them.

- **For example:** a kitchen counter that gathers mail and miscellaneous items, or a chair in the bedroom that gets piled up with clothes. Spend a few minutes clearing this space methodically.

The One-in-one-out rule – for every new item you bring into your home, remove one existing item.

- **For example**: if you buy a new pair of shoes, find an old pair you can donate. This helps to maintain the balance of items in your home and prevents new clutter from accumulating.

The five-minute pick-up: Set a timer for five minutes, and pick up and put away as many out-of-place items as you can. Focus on visible areas that will make the most noticeable impact.

- **For example**: the kitchen counter, the hall table, and the living room floor.

Now, let's take a look at Marie Kondo, the Japanese organizing consultant and author of *The Life-Changing Magic of Tidying Up*. She has become a global phenomenon with her unique approach to decluttering and organizing. Her method, known as the 'KonMari Method,' is detailed and thoughtful and aims to transform not only your space but also your relationship with your belongings.

Here are the fundamental principles of the KonMari Method:

- Commit yourself to tidying up. Successful decluttering requires a genuine commitment to the process. Make a firm decision to start and follow through, and understand that this is more than just organizing your space; it's about creating a whole lifestyle change.
- Visualize your ideal lifestyle. A clear vision of your ideal life and home provides motivation and direction. Think about why and what you want to declutter and how it will improve your life. Write down or create a vision board of your goals and desired living space.

- Focus on discarding first. By doing this first, you will be able to see exactly how much storage space you need and ensure you only keep what truly matters.

The KonMari Categories

Marie Kondo's method involves decluttering by category, not by location. This helps you see the totality of your belongings so that you can make more informed decisions. The categories should be tackled in a specific order:

Clothes

Starting with clothes is often easier because there is usually a less intense emotional attachment to clothing.

- Gather all your clothing from every part of the house and pile it in one place.
- Pick up each item and ask yourself if it 'sparks joy'. Sparking joy means that an item brings a sense of happiness, positivity, or excitement when you pick it up.
- Keep only the items that elicit a joyful response and discard the rest.
- Organize the remaining clothes by type and store them in a way that is easily visible and accessible.

Books

- Books can accumulate quickly and often hold sentimental value, making them harder to part with.
- Collect all your books in one area.
- Handle each book individually and ask yourself if it sparks joy.

- Keep only the books that truly resonate with you. Don't feel obligated to keep books you haven't read or don't intend to re-read.
- Store books upright on shelves with the spines facing outward.

Papers

- Paper clutter can be overwhelming and energy-sucking.
- Gather all papers, including receipts, bills and documents.
- Sort into three categories – pending (needs action), important (needs to be kept), and discard (no longer needed).
- Recycle the 'discard' pile and organize the essential papers in a filing system that is simple and accessible, or else scan and digitize these documents to reduce physical clutter.

Komono (Miscellaneous items)

- This category includes various household items that can easily become cluttered.
- Break this category into sub-categories such as kitchen items, bathroom items, gadgets, etc.
- Handle each item and ask if it sparks joy or serves a genuinely useful purpose.
- Discard duplicates and items that are no longer needed or used.

Sentimental items

- Sentimental items are the hardest to part with and should be addressed last to ensure you have refined your decision-making skills.

- Gather all sentimental items like photos, letters and mementoes.
- Handle each item and ask if it sparks joy. Keep only those items that bring happiness and fond memories.
- Store sentimental items in a dedicated space that honors their importance—for example, creating a memory box for treasured photos and letters, or displaying a few meaningful mementoes where you can see them daily.

This technique has been extremely popular, and with good reason. However, there is a danger for people with ADHD that enthusiastically piling an enormous heap of clothes on the bed or books in the living room will rapidly lead to task paralysis and overwhelm and become a doom pile of its own. It's best, therefore, to break down these tasks by sub-categorizing. For example, instead of tackling all your clothes at once, you could start with your coats or jackets or have a sort-through of all your shoes. For the papers, start with one desk or drawer rather than dealing with all the documents at once. In the kitchen, tackle one counter or cupboard at a time.

Both systems encourage mindfulness about new items and use a one-in-one-out rule to prevent clutter from re-accumulating. It's also important to embrace imperfection and understand that a perfectly organized home at all times isn't realistic. Aim for progress, not perfection, and focus on creating a liveable, functional space rather than an Instagram-perfect, minimalist room. This is the best way to keep the organization on track and avoid overwhelm.

The 'Full Hands' Rule

Another way of keeping clutter at bay with minimum effort is to make it a rule never to leave a room empty handed – because there will always be something in a room that needs to be taken elsewhere. So for example, if you are in the living room and heading to the kitchen and you see that there's an old coffee cup on the side table, don't leave the room without taking it with you; if you are heading from the bedroom to the bathroom, pick up the dirty clothes and toss them in the laundry basket as you go. Always leave a room with full hands. This rule maximizes the efficiency of your movements, and makes sure that every trip out of a room is as productive as possible. It encourages you to be mindful of your surroundings, and helps to prevent mess from piling up.

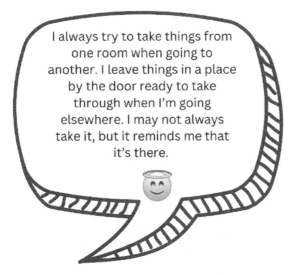

I always try to take things from one room when going to another. I leave things in a place by the door ready to take through when I'm going elsewhere. I may not always take it, but it reminds me that it's there.

One final tip, for those who are financially able and wish to do a big clear-out, hiring a dump trailer can be a great way to get started. They normally have a week-long deadline, which will keep you on track and act as motivation to keep going. You will love how easy it is to dispose of items in the trailer, and it speeds up the whole process. It can even become quite addictive to chuck things away: each space you clear releases another hit of dopamine and creates a lighter, clearer atmosphere in your home.

CHAPTER 10
CLEAN HOUSE, CLEAR MIND

Congratulations, you've done the heavy lifting of decluttering, you've made the hard decisions, said goodbye to the stuff you no longer need, and created some much-needed space. So what's next? It's time to talk about cleaning, and keeping your newly-decluttered spaces clean and clear.

While decluttering is all about making decisions, purging and organizing, cleaning is about maintenance. It's about making sure that the spaces we've worked so hard to declutter remain clean and pleasant to live in. Over the next few chapters, we are going to take a deep dive into how to declutter and clean different areas of the house, but firstly, let's look at what you need to get started.

Cleaning supplies are our tools here, and we need to have the right ones at hand. It's a really good idea to have a core set of basic cleaning supplies stored in every room – especially the kitchen, bathroom, bedroom and living room – so that you don't get stuck on a task because of a lack of cleaning materials close at hand, and you can grab them quickly whenever you have motivation to do a 5-minute sprint.

Cleaning Supplies Checklist

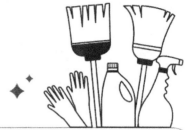

- All-purpose cleaner in a handy spray bottle.
- Glass cleaner for windows, mirrors and shiny surfaces.
- White vinegar in a spray bottle. This is great for streaks on glass, but also for getting out stubborn odors such as pets and cigarettes.
- A spray bottle of degreaser for the kitchen.
- Disinfectant wipes, useful for quick clean-ups; it's good to have packets of these wipes handy in the bathroom and on the kitchen counters.
- Wet & Forget weekly shower cleaner that you spray, leave & rinse off.
- Microfiber cloths, great for dusting and polishing.
- A small, rechargeable hand-held vacuum cleaner. Getting out a big vacuum cleaner from a cluttered cupboard can be overwhelming and lead to task paralysis, so for smaller jobs, a hand-held vacuum that rests on a counter-top is easier to grab and reduces the resistance to making a start.
- A dustpan and brush; great for a quick sweep of the kitchen floor.
- Mop and bucket for washing hardwood, vinyl and tiled floors.
- Dual sponges with a wire wool side and a sponge side are good for tougher spots.
- A plastic scraper is useful for dealing with tough dried-on food.
- Trash bags – always have a good supply.

I do a lot of my cleaning between tasks. I work from home, so for instance when I'm waiting for my lunch to heat up, I'll pick something to clean. I'm always surprised how much I can get done in two minutes. Other times I will tidy the kitchen counter or wipe off the cupboard doors while the kettle is boiling. I don't spend too long on it, but it always makes a difference.

The 'Wipe Down While you Wait' Trick

One of the best ways to fit in a 5-minute burst of cleaning is the 'wipe down while you wait' technique. This makes use of those otherwise 'dead' moments in the kitchen when you are waiting for your meal to warm through or the kettle to boil. See how much you can get done in the 5 minutes it takes for the microwave to heat your meal and for the food to cool down so that it won't burn your mouth. You'll be surprised at what you can achieve in that otherwise dead time: unloading the dishwasher, taking out the trash, wiping down a kitchen counter. And you can do the same during the commercial breaks when you are watching your favorite TV show.

Top 10 Cleaning Hacks

Here's a list of 10 great cleaning hacks to help you keep the house clean with minimum effort:

- Always clean from top to bottom. Dust and dirt fall, so you want to make sure you don't have to clean twice.
- Dry to wet – start with dry cleaning such as dusting and sweeping, then move to wet chores such as mopping and wiping.
- Dust with dryer sheets. Use dryer sheets to dust your surfaces, electronics, blinds, baseboards and ornaments. They pick up much more dust than traditional dusters, and leave behind a pleasant scent. They also leave a trace of anti-static residue which is an effective dust repellent.
- Before cleaning the microwave, place a bowl of water with a slice of lemon in it and heat for two minutes. The steam loosens the grime, making it easier to clean.
- Keep a squeegee in the shower and use it to wipe down the glass walls and doors after each use. It's a quick job that helps to prevent limescale, water spots and soap scum build-up.
- Keep disinfectant wipes in the bathroom for a quick wipe of the sink, faucet and toilet seat each day. Regular wiping off can eliminate the need for a deep clean.
- Do the vacuuming before dusting, as vacuums often churn up dust that gets sent into the air and rests on your surfaces. A lint roller can be great for picking up dust on difficult surfaces such as lampshades, upholstered furniture and even car seats.
- When you are putting away groceries, try to clear one shelf of the refrigerator and use a cloth to wipe it down before

you fill it with your food items. It keeps the interior of the refrigerator clean without massive effort.

- Use a toothbrush for small crevices. An old toothbrush is perfect for cleaning small, hard-to-reach areas like grout lines and around faucets. Just dip it into some cleaning fluid, or a mix of vinegar and baking soda, and scrub.
- Pre-treat stains immediately. Keep a small spray bottle of stain remover handy, so that whenever a spill or stain happens, you are ready to blitz it straight away. This will help prevent you having to scrub and treat set-in stains later.

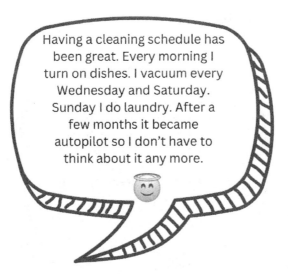

Establishing Regular Habits

One of the most important things with regards to cleaning is regularity and consistency. The more regularly you clean, the less you will need to do the dreaded 'deep clean' which is a bigger beast altogether.

Having a cleaning schedule can really help: knowing that on Mondays you do the vacuuming, Tuesdays it's the bathroom and Wednesdays the kitchen counters can really help to keep you on track.

By regularly wiping down surfaces and minimizing the build-up of dust and grime, taking just five minutes here and five minutes there, you will need less time and effort to keep the house clean. It's so much easier to add one more step to a job you are already winning at, than starting a whole new task. Having said that, we all know that life happens, and if you can't clean at all for a time, don't stress. Just pick up where you left off when you have more motivation and energy. And don't forget to celebrate each win and give yourself rewards. Acknowledging your efforts is so important in helping to stay motivated.

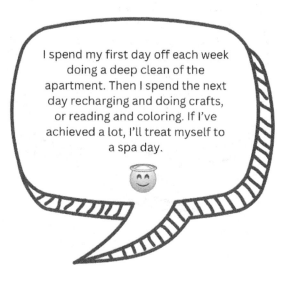

I spend my first day off each week doing a deep clean of the apartment. Then I spend the next day recharging and doing crafts, or reading and coloring. If I've achieved a lot, I'll treat myself to a spa day.

Deep Breath – the Deep Clean

Have a look at these tips for starting your deep clean.

TIPS FOR STARTING YOUR DEEP CLEAN

 1. Make a checklist for each room, and put the tasks that need the most attention at the top of the list.

 2. Gather all your supplies so that you have everything easily to hand. Invest in good-quality cleaning tools and products that will make the task easier.

 3. Pick one section of a room to work on at a time to avoid overwhelm. That way, even if you don't complete a whole room in one session, you will still have made a great start.

 4. Set a timer for 5 minutes to get going, then take a break if you need. Keep working for a maximum of 35 minutes and take a longer break when the time is up.

 5. Podcasts, audio books, music and your favorite TV shows are your friends here. It's a lot more fun to clean when you have 'The Simpsons', Beyoncé or a gripping audio book on in the background to keep you company. It's almost as good as having a body double.

 6. Body doubling apps and websites can help by matching you up with another person online who is also working on a task. You keep each other accountable for an hour of focused work.

Here's a run-down of the main tasks for each room. Of course, you may have others that you can add, but it's sometimes helpful to have a basic overview of the most important tasks.

Kitchen

- Do a thorough clean of the inside of the refrigerator and freezer: take all food items out and wipe down all shelves and surfaces with warm water and baking soda.
- Clean the oven, stovetop and microwave.
- Clean all the countertops and backsplash.
- Scrub the sink and clean the area around the faucets. Pour a half cup of baking soda down the drain, followed by a half cup of vinegar. Let it fizz for a few minutes, then flush it down with hot water. This will help keep the drain clear.
- Sweep and mop the floor.
- Empty out cabinets and drawers and wipe down the inside surfaces.
- Run a clean cycle on the dishwasher and washing machine

Living Room

- Shampoo the carpets and wash the curtains. Consider renting a steam cleaner once a year for this job.
- Clean the blinds. Slip an old sock onto your hand, dip it in a mixture of equal parts vinegar and water and run your hand along the slats of the blinds to remove dust and grime.
- Vacuum behind and under furniture.
- Wipe the baseboards with a damp cloth or a dryer sheet, to repel dust.

- Clean and dust fan blades – use an old pillowcase to slip over the fan blade and pull it back to catch all the dust and prevent it falling into the room.

Bathroom

- Scrub the shower and tub and clean grout lines and areas around the faucet with an old toothbrush.
- Clean the inside bowl of the toilet with a toilet brush, and give the seat, lid and handle a wipe with disinfectant wipes.
- Scrub the sink and countertop and clean mirrors with glass cleaner to remove water spots.
- Mop the floor, especially the area around the sink and toilet.

Bedroom

- Wash all bedding, sheets, pillowcases etc. Wash and tumble dry pillows and comforters.
- Vacuum the mattress and spot-clean any stains. Consider using a mattress protector to keep it clean.
- Dust all surfaces including night stands, shelves and cupboards, light fittings and ceiling fans.
- Vacuum under the bed and other furniture.

Let's talk About Body Doubling

One of the most effective ways to help you get started and keep going with a big cleaning project is body doubling. This is a strategy where you have another person physically present to help you stay focused and motivated. They don't necessarily have to be doing the same task as you and they don't even need to be in the same room as you – the idea is that their presence increases your accountability and makes it harder to get distracted. Your body double can be a friend, family member, someone on the end of a phone line, or even someone you've found through an online community. The key is to have someone there to help you stay on track.

This is a game-changer for some people. There's something about the low-level social accountability that just clicks. Having another person there increases the feeling of being monitored, making it harder to get distracted. Even if your body double is just chilling and watching TV while you are cleaning up the kitchen, their presence somehow makes it easier to resist the constant urge to abandon ship.

Of course, it's even better when they roll up their sleeves and work alongside you. This creates a sense of shared purpose and motivation to stay on task, which can be much more fun and rewarding than doing it alone. It's like having a teammate in your corner, cheering you on and helping you stay focused.

Body doubling can take place online, with apps such as Dubbii (https://www.dubbii.app) Deepwrk (https://www.deepwrk.io), RescueTime (https://www.rescuetime.com) and Flow Club (https://www.flow.club) that connect adults with ADHD in an online community. Your online body double will act as your co-worker or decluttering buddy, and you can also use the gamification tools and guided focus sessions to help get you motivated, escape distractions and stay on target.

Sharing your cleaning and decluttering successes with others can also amplify their impact. Whether it's posting before-and-after pictures of your newly-organized space on social media or simply telling a friend about your progress, sharing can reinforce your sense of achievement. It also allows you to celebrate together, multiplying the joy of your successes. Plus, sharing your journey can inspire others to embark on their own organizational efforts, spreading the positive vibes even further.

We've Got to the End of Part 1

So, here we are already at the end of part 1. What have we learned so far? Well, we've established the basics. We've looked at some of the myths and misconceptions about ADHD and some of the unique challenges that people with ADHD face. We've worked out what kind of organization methods might work best for you, and most importantly, we have talked about the power of the five-minute task for beating procrastination and building momentum. We've looked at lots of ways of tackling the twin monsters of decluttering and cleaning, and we know what tools we need. We now have a really good idea of how to make a start.

In the second part of this book, we're going to take a deep-dive into some of the main areas of the house – the kitchen, bedroom, living room and so on, so that you can apply what you have already learned to specific areas of the home. We'll also be looking at ways of clearing the digital clutter, great tips for meal planning and grocery shopping and how to inspire kids to tidy their spaces. See you there!

MAKE A DIFFERENCE WITH YOUR REVIEW

"I think we forget sometimes how blessed we are to be able to help others and make a difference!"

— GAUTAM RODE

Dear Reader,

You know that profound sense of satisfaction you feel after helping someone? That incredible feeling of knowing you've made a difference in someone's life?

Today, I have an important request for you...

Imagine helping someone who, like you, sometimes feels overwhelmed with the clutter and chaos of everyday life, particularly because they have ADHD. They aspire to create a more organized and peaceful environment but are unsure where to start.

You have already taken an important step towards this goal by buying and reading this book, and I hope with all my heart that you are finding it helpful so far. But there are many more people out there who are still struggling.

My mission in writing 'Stress-Free Organizing with ADHD' is to assist as many people with ADHD as possible to improve their lives by giving them a roadmap towards organization and self-care. To achieve this, I need to amplify the reach of this book to as many people as possible.

This is where your support becomes crucial. Many people decide to read a book based on the experiences and recommendations of others. Therefore, I'm asking for your assistance in a way that can make a significant difference:

Could you leave a review for this book?

It requires only a moment of your time, but your words could profoundly impact someone else's life. Your review could help someone like you to find order in their life by taking the first simple, easy steps laid out in this book.

To leave your review on Amazon, please scan the QR code below:

By leaving a review, you are joining a community of individuals dedicated to making a positive difference. Your contribution is invaluable, and together, we can help others with ADHD achieve a more organized and fulfilling life.

Thank you sincerely for your support. Let's continue the journey towards creating a clearer, calmer and happier space together.

With gratitude,
Caroline Singer

CHAPTER 11

LET'S START WITH THE KITCHEN

The kitchen is the heart of every home, where we cook, eat, socialize and sometimes even work. It can feel like a never-ending task to keep it clean, because nine times out of ten it's also the most cluttered room of the house, with piles of dirty dishes, unsorted mail, household miscellany and food packaging. So it's probably the first place to spark feelings of overwhelm and task paralysis. The sheer number and volume of items to clean and clear seems overwhelming, and the complexity of the task, with so many different steps, can lead to procrastination and feelings of stress.

The very best way to kickstart your kitchen decluttering and cleaning is by setting yourself a time to start. For example, set an alarm on your phone and tell yourself that at 10.30 on the dot you are going to make a start on the kitchen. Promise yourself that you only have to do the minimum of 5 minutes of cleaning. Begin by focusing on what you can see. It's all about getting instant gratification that fuels further action. Grab your 'keep', 'discard' and 'trash' boxes and set a timer. Commit to spending five minutes doing a sweep of the countertops. This is a great place to start, because clear surfaces look instantly better and give you space to prepare meals without having to shove aside a mountain of miscellaneous items first. Anything that doesn't belong on the counter, either because it's not frequently used or because it's just out of place, goes into one of the boxes. If you're unsure, use the 'Maybe' box. Right now, it's about clearing the visual clutter. You'll be amazed at how much of a difference just five minutes can make. Clearing your counters provides an immediate visual relief and a sense of accomplishment that's incredibly motivating.

Quick Wins in the Kitchen That Can Be Tackled in 5-Minute Sprints

Once you've cleared the counters and if you have motivation to continue, look for other quick wins. These tasks are small enough to tackle in short bursts but impactful enough to make a noticeable difference. How about those dishes? Fill the sink with lots of hot water and washing-up liquid, turn the music up, and set yourself a challenge of washing up as many pans, mugs, and dishes as you can in 5 minutes. Once you get going, you'll be amazed at how fast you can do it.

Now think about organizing one of the drawers, and ask the question of each item – is it genuinely useful and functional, or does it make you smile? If not, discard it. Organize the remaining kitchen utensils by usage frequency, storing everyday items within easy reach and less-used items in less accessible spaces.

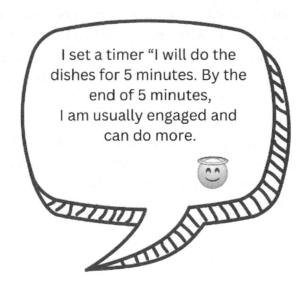

Other tasks in the kitchen, such as tidying a pantry shelf, clearing out expired items in the refrigerator, or cleaning the oven, can be done in about five minutes, and each task you do leaves one less corner of chaos in your kitchen. The trick is to keep it simple and specific. Set a timer and go! You'll find that these mini decluttering and cleaning sprints add up quickly, significantly reducing the overall clutter in your kitchen. Here are some more ideas for quick 5-minute tasks that will help you keep your kitchen clean and manageable.

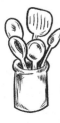

5-Minute Wins in the Kitchen

Quick and easy 5-minute tasks that make a big impact.

- Wipe down the countertops. Keep a pack of antiseptic wipes handy on the counter.

- Sweep the floor - take 5 minutes to clear away crumbs & dust.

- Take out the trash or recycling.

- Put away clean dishes drying on the rack.

- Fill the sink with hot water and washing up liquid and do the dishes - or put them in to soak so they're on their way to being clean.

- Clear and wipe the dining table.

- Pick one shelf in the pantry and throw out expired items.

- Wipe clean the appliances – toaster, coffee maker, microwave etc.

Simple, Maintainable Systems for Keeping the Kitchen Organized

Now, let's talk systems. In the long run, the key to keeping your kitchen clean and clutter-free is to implement simple organizing systems that you can maintain easily. This doesn't mean you need an elaborate set-up worthy of a home magazine. Instead, focus on functional, easy-to-maintain solutions.

- Use drawer dividers for utensils so that everything has a place and you don't end up with a jumbled mess.
- Invest in clear containers and hanging pockets for your pantry to keep food items visible and accessible.
- Label shelves in the fridge to designate areas for condiments, drinks, leftovers, etc.
- Place a box or basket in a prominent place on the kitchen counter or table, as a 'drop zone' for all the papers, letters, bills and school circulars that otherwise get left lying around.

These simple systems are effective and will give you the confidence that you can maintain order day after day.

My antibacterial wipes live on my kitchen countertop so that I can do a quick wipe-down every morning while I'm waiting for the kettle to boil. Then every Friday I use the degreaser spray to wipe all my cupboards, counters and backsplash to clean up the week's cooking grime.

The One-Minute Rule

Maintaining the tidiness of your kitchen is all about incorporating small habits into your daily routine that prevent clutter from building up again. One effective habit is the "one-minute rule"—if a task can be done in one minute or less, do it immediately. This could be anything from putting the spices back in the rack after cooking to hanging up the dish towel instead of leaving it on the counter. Additionally, make it a practice to do a quick sweep of the kitchen each night, resetting any areas that have become disorganized throughout the day. These quick daily resets help keep your kitchen looking consistently clean and make the space more enjoyable to use.

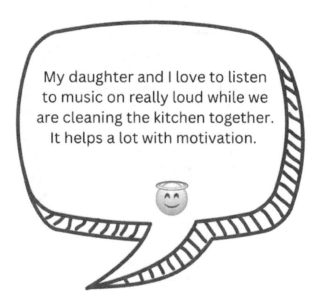

My daughter and I love to listen to music on really loud while we are cleaning the kitchen together. It helps a lot with motivation.

Create a 'Drop Zone'

Another great tip is to get yourself a basket, file sorter or box file for the kitchen 'drop zone', where all the bills, unopened mail, school circulars and other documents go to die. Place the box or basket in a prominent position that is easy for everyone to access. Then you and the rest of the family can simply drop all documents, mail and other papers in there so that they will not get lost. Spend a few minutes once a week sorting through the box, recycling or shredding the papers you don't need, and dealing with the important stuff before it gets out of date.

By following these steps, you can transform your kitchen from a clutter hotspot to a streamlined space that supports your daily life. Remember, the goal isn't perfection but functionality and ease. So, take a deep breath, set your timer, and get ready for your kitchen to become not just a place where you cook, but a space where creativity and calm coexist beautifully. And don't forget to reward yourself when you're done!

CHAPTER 12

LIVING ROOM ORGANIZATION: QUICK WINS FOR A COSY SPACE

Ah, the living room – that multi-functional hub where you chill, chat, binge-watch, and regularly trip over a random collection of toys, shoes and other stuff that definitely shouldn't be there. Let's make it a space that invites calm and cosiness rather than chaos and clutter.

First up, identify your focus areas. Where does the doom pile of clutter tend to accumulate? Maybe it's the stacks of magazines and mail on the coffee table or the remote controls and gaming gadgets sprawled across the sofa. Or perhaps it's the shoes and bags that seem to have taken up permanent residence around your couch. Pinpointing these hotspots gives you a clear target for your quick decluttering missions.

Once you've identified these zones, it's all about quick clears. This isn't the time to sort through every single magazine with the precision of an archaeologist. Instead, set the timer and challenge yourself to make rapid-fire decisions. Throw out all the trash for an easy win, then decide whether to keep, toss, or donate – go with your gut and move fast. If it hasn't been used in months or doesn't bring you joy, it's time to say goodbye.

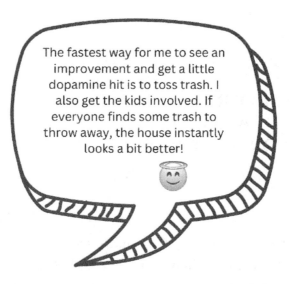

The fastest way for me to see an improvement and get a little dopamine hit is to toss trash. I also get the kids involved. If everyone finds some trash to throw away, the house instantly looks a bit better!

Now, let's talk about one of the simplest yet most effective hacks for keeping your living room tidy: boxes and baskets. These aren't just containers; they're your clutter-busting allies. Choose a couple of stylish baskets or nicely-decorated boxes that complement your décor and use them to corral the most important and frequently-used items. This strategy isn't just about storage but accessibility and ease. When everything has a designated home, consider what to do with the rest of the stuff that doesn't fit into the storage boxes. Either donate or throw them out.

Once you have freed up some floor and surface space, and if you still have motivation and energy, set a timer and do a quick vacuum and wipe down surfaces with a duster or damp cloth. This will help to freshen up the room and makes a big difference to the feeling of cleanliness. Clutter and dust are huge energy-suckers, and it's amazing how much the atmosphere of a room changes for the better when it is not only clutter-free but also clean.

I tell myself I don't need to tidy up the whole living room, I just have to tidy the coffee table, and a lot of times that leads me to doing more. For me, it's about breaking a task up into something smaller and then getting started, with the expectation that just starting a tiny bit is actually good enough.

Creating a relaxing environment goes beyond decluttering; it's also about setting a vibe. Consider the arrangement of your furniture – does it promote ease of movement, or does it contribute to the clutter? Sometimes, simply rearranging your setup can significantly enhance the flow and feel of the room. Get the family involved in a spot of reorganization. Aim for an open, inviting layout that discourages clutter accumulation. Position seating to foster conversation and cosiness. Incorporate soft lighting to enhance the ambience – think lamps with warm bulbs rather than harsh overhead lights. These touches encourage relaxation and make your living room a true retreat from the hustle and bustle of daily life.

Lastly, implementing a five-minute daily maintenance routine can work wonders. This isn't about deep cleaning; it's more like a quick tidy-up to reset the space each day. Spend five minutes each evening clearing surfaces, fluffing cushions, and returning any out-of-place items to their rightful homes. This daily habit keeps your living room looking great and makes it a more enjoyable space for unwinding at the end of the day. Think of it as a gift to yourself and your family – a serene space to greet you every morning and welcome you back every evening.

By focusing on these critical areas, using intelligent storage solutions, creating a cosy layout, and maintaining the space with simple daily routines, you can transform your living room into a haven of peace and relaxation. So, take a moment, look around, and start envisioning your living room not just as it is but as it could be – a beautiful, calm, clutter-free space.

CHAPTER 13

TRANSFORMING YOUR BEDROOM INTO A HAVEN IN MINUTES

I magine stepping into your bedroom after a long, bustling day. Does the room invite calm and relaxation, or does it give you a sinking feeling and a reminder of all the chores that await? A bedroom's ambience can significantly impact your sleep quality and stress levels, transforming it from merely a place to sleep into a sanctuary of serenity. For those who are navigating life with ADHD, and for whom winding down can often feel like a task in its own right, a clutter-free and well-organized bedroom becomes not just a luxury but a necessity.

The importance of maintaining a peaceful bedroom extends beyond aesthetics. Clutter is a visual and mental irritant, draining our energy and keeping our minds in a state of low-level stress. It's like background noise that you don't notice until it stops. By decluttering your bedroom, you have a space where you can effectively turn off this noise, allowing your mind to relax and prepare for rest. Set the timer to 5 minutes and start with visible surfaces like nightstands and dressers. Clear off anything that is obviously trash or doesn't belong in the bedroom —random receipts, old coffee cups, last week's laundry that never made it to the closet. Even these minor adjustments can make a big difference in shifting your room's atmosphere from chaotic to calm.

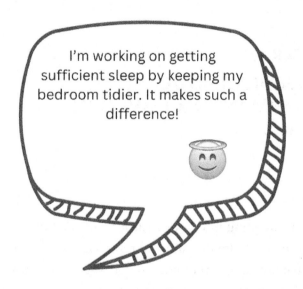

Now, for some more quick wins that can transform your bedroom without needing to block off an entire weekend. Begin with the floor around your bedside area—often a hotspot for miscellaneous items to accumulate. Spend just five minutes clearing out old magazines, unused gadgets, or trinkets that have lost their significance. Next, take another five minutes to tackle under the bed. This often-forgotten space can be a breeding ground for dust and long-lost items. Clearing it out not only provides additional storage space but also contributes to your room's overall cleanliness and energy. How about the 'floordrobe' – that trail of clothes cluttering up the floor? Set the timer and challenge yourself to scoop up as many clothes as you can in five minutes, dropping the dirty clothes into the laundry basket and leaving the rest next to the closet to be hung up when you have the motivation.

Tackling the Closet

Now, how about that closet? This can often be a daunting task, but breaking it down into small, manageable chunks can make even this Big Daddy of a job more achievable. Start by setting clear goals. Do you want to create more room in the closet or a better system for storing your clothes?

Secondly, identify tasks that will take just 5 minutes and make all the difference.

- Start by gathering and removing all the empty hangers. This will instantly give you more space and a clearer view of what's in the closet.
- Next, grab any clothes that need washing and put them into the laundry basket.
- Then, you could start sorting through your accessories – belts, scarves, hats, etc. Quickly go through these items, deciding what to keep, donate or throw away.
- Spend a few minutes pairing up shoes and lining them neatly or placing them in a hanging organizer.
- While doing that, you can decide whether to keep or donate any shoes you haven't worn for a while.

Then you can start sorting your clothing. But don't try and do it all in one rush. Focus on one category at a time – underwear, t-shirts, sweaters, etc. Perhaps do one or two categories per day, so that you don't end up creating huge mounds of clothes that could become new doom piles of their own.

HOW TO SORT CLOTHES

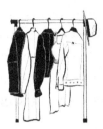

 Pick up each item one by one, and ask yourself if you have worn it in the past year, if it brings you joy, and if it goes with anything else in your closet.

 If you are undecided, you can try an item of clothing on and ask yourself 'do I like the way I feel in this?' If not, it can go.

 Check for any clothes that you want to keep, but that need minor repairs (missing buttons, small tears, or stains) and set them aside to fix later or take to the dry cleaners.

 Look out for fabrics that are heavily pilled, elastic that has lost its mojo, any clothes that have stains you can't get out, or tears that are unfixable. They are an instant 'throw'.

 Donate clothes you have hardly ever worn, and please don't feel guilty about it: you will be giving someone else the chance to enjoy an item that looked great in the store but didn't quite suit you enough in real life.

Once you can see the floor again, and the shelves are clear, and if you have energy and motivation to spare, you can vacuum or sweep the floor of your closet and wipe down the surfaces to remove dust. These quick tasks, achievable in short bursts, reduce overwhelm and create visible results that turn your closet into a space you can enjoy rather than dread. Now, take a break and give yourself a reward. You deserve it!

Lastly, incorporating a nightly reset routine can really enhance the tranquility of your bedroom. This doesn't need to be a lengthy process; just a few minutes each evening can maintain the order and comfort of your space. This might include tasks like folding blankets, plumping pillows, placing clothes in a laundry basket or back in the closet, and setting your shoes neatly aside. It's also an excellent time to prepare for the next day. Lay out your clothes, refill your water bottle, or set out any items you need for the morning. This helps keep your bedroom tidy and sets you up for a smoother start the next day.

CHAPTER 14

LAUNDRY MADE EASY: SMALL STEPS TO BIG IMPACT

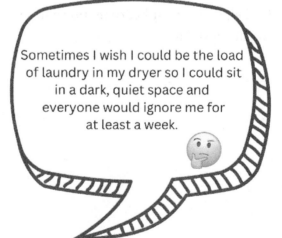

Sometimes I wish I could be the load of laundry in my dryer so I could sit in a dark, quiet space and everyone would ignore me for at least a week.

I f the mere mention of laundry has you envisioning an endless cycle of wash, dry, fold, repeat, you're not alone. For those living with ADHD, managing the laundry can often feel like trying to tame a beast that grows two heads for every one you cut off. Let's break down the laundry process into manageable steps, making it less of a chore and more of a triumph.

Simplifying the Laundry Process

Laundry becomes a lot less daunting when you break the process down into smaller, more digestible steps. For starters, separate your laundry tasks into distinct stages—sorting, washing, drying, folding, ironing and putting away. Tackle each stage separately and give yourself permission to pause in between. For instance, today, you could sort the laundry into different piles—whites, colors, delicates. Tomorrow, tackle washing the whites. This approach makes the laundry feel less overwhelming and allows you to focus fully on one manageable task at a time, reducing the likelihood of ADHD-induced overwhelm.

5-Minute Laundry Tasks

Now, let's sprinkle some magic into the mix with 5-minute tasks. Here are a few suggestions for breaking down the laundry into smaller, more manageable chunks that can help you keep on top of it. Set a timer for five minutes and see how much you can get done. You will be surprised at how a few minutes here and there can add up to a lot of progress.

5-minute Laundry Tasks

- Sorting Laundry: Separate your clothes into different piles—whites, darks, and colors—plus a pile for delicate items. This helps to streamline the washing process.

- Treating stains: Spend a few minutes applying stain remover on your clothes before putting them in the wash.

- Starting a wash cycle: Load your sorted laundry into the washing machine, add detergent and start the wash cycle.

- Folding clothes: Grab a small batch of clean clothes and fold them. This might include towels, t-shirts, and socks.

- Hanging clothes: Spend 5 minutes hanging items that need to air dry, or that should be stored on hangers, e.g. dresses, shirts & pants.

- Emptying the lint trap in your dryer: A quick but essential task which improves efficiency and reduces the risk of fire.

- Putting away laundry: If you have a few clean items left out, spend a few minutes putting them away in drawers or closets.

- Prepping items for dry cleaning: If you have garments that need dry cleaning, use a few minutes to gather and bag them for your next trip to the cleaners.

Creating a Laundry Schedule

One of the secrets to keeping on top of laundry is to create and stick to a schedule. This might sound a bit daunting, but establishing a routine – say, washing clothes on Tuesday evenings and Saturday mornings – can help turn an erratic chore into a predictable, manageable part of your week. A schedule takes the guesswork out of the equation. No more standing in front of the washing machine, wondering if you should throw in a load. You know precisely when and what you'll be washing, making it easier to plan and stay on track. Tell the family about it, so that they know to bring down their laundry baskets on the right day. Regular laundry days prevent the pile from becoming a mountain. Before it gets out of hand, you're already on top of it.

Organizational Tools for Laundry

Lastly, let's talk tools, because it's worth investing in a few key organizational tools to make the laundry process smoother. If you have space, multiple hampers or bins are really helpful – use them to pre-sort laundry by color, fabric type, or cleaning method right from the get-go. This saves time on sorting day and keeps everything neatly contained. For those pesky missing socks, have a small bin or bag where single socks can wait to be reunited with their partners. Also, folding boards can dramatically speed up the folding process and make your clothes look neatly pressed without needing to iron them.

By integrating these strategies—breaking down the process into stages, tackling quick tasks, sticking to a schedule, and using the right tools—you can transform how you handle laundry. With these steps, you'll keep your laundry in check and free up mental and physical space for more enjoyable activities.

CHAPTER 15

ORGANIZING WITH YOUR CHILD'S MIND IN MIND

Tidying up a child's room can often feel like trying to organize a bag of confetti post-pop —especially when you bring the little ones into the equation. The trick? Get them involved early and make it fun! Remember, kids are keen observers and natural mimickers. They watch you more closely than you might think, absorbing your habits and attitudes like little sponges. That's why leading by example isn't just a phrase— it's one of your most powerful tools in teaching organization. Let your kids see you making your bed, sorting the mail, or putting things back where they belong. Over time, these actions set a visual standard for what organization looks like.

I've started doing these 5-minute clean-ups with the kids. It's been a total game-changer! I set a timer for 5 minutes and we all pitch in for a short burst. The key is, I'm working right alongside them. Each kid gets their own zone to focus on, and I got them their own mini broom and dustpan. After just 10 minutes of us all working together, we can get the whole house looking presentable again.

Engaging younger children in the organization process starts with turning clean-up time into a game. Who can sort their toys the fastest? You can set a timer and challenge them to beat the clock. The key is to inject a sense of play and competition, which makes the task more enjoyable and taps into children's natural love for games. Offer small rewards like an extra bedtime story, a favorite snack, or a special sticker. You could also use music during clean-up times. Playing upbeat songs can turn chore time into a dance party. This approach keeps them engaged and helps them associate positive feelings with organization, which is crucial for developing long-term tidying habits.

For older children and teens, you might involve them in tasks such as setting the table or sorting laundry by color. Set up a challenge: who can declutter their room and keep it tidy for a whole week? These tasks give them a clear role and responsibility, which can be both empowering and educational. Don't forget to build in a rewards system. It's crucial, too, to keep these tasks age-appropriate. Expecting too much too soon can lead to frustration on both sides. Be patient and celebrate their efforts, not just the outcomes. This encouragement reinforces their desire to help and builds their confidence in handling responsibilities.

Creating Simple, Kid-Friendly Systems

When it comes to systems, simplicity is your best friend. Kids require precise, straightforward organization methods that they can easily understand and follow. Start by introducing zones in their room: one for play, one for sleep, and one for study. Use visual labels with pictures for younger children who can't yet read. For example, open shelving and bins with a picture of a car for toy cars, or a clear plastic box with a picture of crayons for art supplies. This helps them understand where things belong and supports their learning and independence in maintaining order. The less complicated the system, the more likely they will use it consistently.

Regular decluttering sessions can also become a norm in your child's routine. Set a regular 'declutter date'—maybe once a month or at the end of each season—where you and your child go through their things together. This is an excellent opportunity to discuss the value of giving and sharing, by encouraging them to donate toys they no longer use or clothes they have outgrown. Make it a celebratory event by marking it on the calendar and maybe following it up with a favorite activity or treat. This keeps their space tidy and teaches them about empathy and generosity. Plus, it helps them decide what items are truly important to them, fostering a sense of responsibility and critical thinking.

Finally, emphasize that what they are doing isn't just about keeping spaces tidy; it's a crucial life skill. Teaching organizational skills to children is an investment in their future. Starting with the basics like putting toys back after playing, or making the bed each morning, you can adapt the tasks as they grow, gradually introducing more complex tasks, such as planning out their school bag the night before or managing a small weekly chore chart.

Acknowledge their efforts and successes along the way; a little praise and a reward can go a long way in building their confidence and motivation. Remember, the goal is to equip them with skills that will serve them throughout life, turning the seemingly mundane task of organizing into a fundamental component of their daily routine.

Tidying up teaches children responsibility, self-reliance, and the importance of caring for their environment. These lessons go beyond the physical spaces; they start to understand how to manage their time, meet their commitments, and respect their belongings and those of others. As they grow, these skills help them navigate schoolwork, friendships, and eventually, their own homes and workspaces.

CHAPTER 16
THE HOME OFFICE: BOOSTING PRODUCTIVITY 5 MINUTES AT A TIME

It's probably true that, at times, your home office feels less like a bastion of productivity and more like a black hole where papers go to get lost and coffee cups come to retire. But you can transform this chaos into a powerhouse of efficiency, all in just five-minute increments. Starting with your desk, the command center of your work universe, let's tackle the clutter that's been doing nothing but eating away at your focus.

Decluttering the Desk

Picture this: a desk that only holds what you need and actually lets you see the surface. Revolutionary, right? Begin by removing everything from your desk. Now, breathe. It's time to rebuild this space piece by piece. Set a timer for five minutes, and challenge yourself to put back only the items you really need – your computer, a notepad for sudden bursts of inspiration, and a pen or two. Next, address the less obvious items. Do you really need six different blocks of sticky notes? Probably not. Spend another few minutes throwing out all the things you do not need. Don't overthink it; act quickly and decisively. Each item you choose to keep should earn its place back on your desk by either being essential for your work, or contributing positively to your workspace environment. This clears physical space and helps minimize mental clutter, allowing you to focus more on the tasks at hand. The rest can be thrown out or donated.

Creating an Environment that Fosters Focus and Productivity

The décor of your workspace can profoundly influence how you feel and perform. Consider the lighting—natural light can boost your mood and energy, so, if possible, position your desk near a window. If natural light isn't an option, opt for soft, warm artificial light rather than harsh overhead fluorescents. Plants are a great addition to a workspace; they purify the air and add life to your environment, making it more enjoyable to spend hours at your desk.

Establishing Short, Daily Routines to Keep the Home Office Organized and Functional

Finally, the key to sustaining this newfound orderliness is routine maintenance. Spend the last five minutes of your workday doing a quick tidy-up. File away papers, clear out your email inbox, and straighten up your desk. As you do this, take a moment to set your goals for the next day. This can be as simple as jotting down the tasks you need to complete or the projects you want to work on. By setting these goals, you're preparing your mind for the next day's work and ensuring you start off on the right foot. This helps keep your space organized and sets you up for a smooth start the following day. Making this a daily habit can transform your end-of-day routine into a resetting ritual, ensuring you leave your workspace feeling accomplished and ready to enjoy your off-the-clock activities without any nagging thoughts of disarray.

Through these simple yet effective strategies, your home office can transition from being a source of stress to a sanctuary of productivity. Just remember, the key isn't to overhaul everything in one go, but to make consistent, small improvements. These incremental changes can dramatically enhance your work environment, allowing you to feel more in control, focused, efficient, and ultimately, successful in your endeavors.

CHAPTER 17

DIGITAL DECLUTTERING: MANAGING EMAILS, FILES AND NOTIFICATIONS

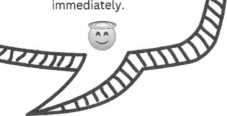

Sorting emails definitely helps me. Work emails manually go to a folder, subscriptions go automatically to separate folders, email receipts/confirmations get a folder, action items get a star - especially if I cannot deal with them immediately.

D o you ever feel like your digital life is just as cluttered as that junk drawer everyone has in their kitchen? You know, the one filled with old batteries, expired coupons, and that random assortment of keys to who-knows-what? Just as a cluttered home can make you feel overwhelmed and scattered, a cluttered digital space can do the same to your mental space. It's time to tackle the digital mess with the same techniques you'd use for that messy drawer.

Strategies for Managing Email Overload Without Getting Overwhelmed

Let's start with your email, which can often feel like a beast forever hungry for more attention. Achieving 'Inbox Zero' — that mythical land where no unread emails dwell — might seem like a fairy tale. But it's actually doable with the right approach.

Here are 6 tips to get you started:

1. First, turn off all email notifications. If there's anything urgent, the sender will text or call you. Give yourself the gift of not being constantly interrupted by new email alerts, especially when you are in the middle of something else. It will also remove the association of emails with a sense of stress.
2. Second, if an email doesn't need a response, archive it straight away.
3. Third, if an email can be answered in under two minutes, do it right away.
4. Fourth, for the emails that need more time, categorize them into three folders: 'Urgent', 'Read Later', or 'Waiting for Response'. This simple act of sorting can make your inbox feel less like a black hole of tasks.

5. Now, think about scheduling a regular 5- or 10-minute email wrap-up session at the end of each day and an 'email hour' each week where you tackle the backlog. It's like setting a date with your inbox; sticking to it can transform your email from foe to friend.

6. If it is easier, and appropriate to the situation, you could consider answering an email with a short video. You'll be surprised by how much information you can communicate in a 30-second iPhone or Loom video that might have taken you an hour to compose in written form.

Creating Intuitive Digital Filing Systems That Reduce Search Time and Increase Efficiency

Next up, let's sort out those digital files. Creating a filing system that mimics your brain's thinking can save you hours of frustrated searching. Start with broad categories that make sense to you—like 'Work', 'Personal', 'Bills', 'Kids' etc.—and then get more specific with subfolders. Be generous with labels and color-coding; visual cues can help guide your ADHD brain straight to the file it seeks. And remember, digital clutter can be just as overwhelming as physical clutter, so make a habit of regularly deleting anything you no longer need.

Now, how about those annoying app notifications that are constantly demanding your attention? It's time to take control. Dive into your phone, tablet, and computer settings, and turn off non-essential notifications. Choose to get updates from only the apps that you deem truly important. For everything else, schedule specific times to check-in. This not only cuts down on distractions, but also helps reduce the anxiety that comes from the constant pings that demand you respond. It's like putting your devices on a 'need to know' basis and trust me; they don't need to know as much as they think they do!

Finally, make digital decluttering a regular part of your routine. Just like your 5-minute cleaning and tidying routines, set aside time for a 5-minute digital cleanup. This could involve clearing out your download folder, organizing your desktop, or unsubscribing from newsletters that you skip over anyway. Regular maintenance keeps everything running smoothly, keeping you in control and less overwhelmed.

CHAPTER 18

THE ART OF THE BRAIN DUMP: CLEARING MENTAL CLUTTER

D o you sometimes feel like you have 2,000 ideas for doing things, want to buy stuff for 200 new projects and start 20 new hobbies, but without actually following through? For those with ADHD, mental clutter often keeps us from focusing on what truly matters. Enter the brain dump, a simple yet revolutionary way to declutter your mind, much like you'd clear out a cluttered drawer.

What is a Brain Dump?

Think of a brain dump as a mental purge, a way to liberate yourself from the swirling thoughts that often keep you from focusing on what truly matters. It's not about organizing thoughts as you go; it's about unleashing them and letting them flow, without judgment or interruption. This process can be incredibly empowering. It reduces the mental overload that often leads to feeling overwhelmed, anxious, or paralyzed by too many thoughts or decisions. By transferring your internal chaos onto paper, you're effectively clearing out the mental space needed to focus on tasks, make decisions, and generally feel less overwhelmed. This simple act can be very helpful, especially before starting a new project, planning your week, or whenever you feel mental fog creeping in.

A Step-by-step Guide to Effectively Performing a Brain Dump

1. Start by grabbing a notebook or opening a new digital document—this will be your mind's playground.
2. Set a timer for 10 to 15 minutes, and just start writing. Write down everything that comes to mind: tasks, worries, ideas, what you need to buy at the grocery store, an email you forgot to send – literally anything and everything.
3. Don't worry about making sense or being neat. The goal is not to create a masterpiece; it's to unload every little thought taking up space in your brain. You might be surprised at what emerges when you give your thoughts free rein.
4. This process is particularly useful on days when you're feeling stuck or when your brain feels like it's on overdrive. It's like taking a broom and sweeping out the dusty corners of your mind.
5. Once everything is on paper, it's time to bring some order to the chaos. Start by looking for themes or categories— perhaps there are several tasks related to a specific project, or multiple worries about an upcoming event. Begin grouping these thoughts together. Use different colored pens or highlighters to categorize them visually.
6. Then, decide on a course of action for each category. What needs immediate attention? What can be scheduled for later? What can be delegated or eliminated? This step transforms your brain dump from a pile of random

thoughts into a structured action plan, making it easier to tackle each item without feeling overwhelmed.

To truly reap the benefits of brain dumping, make it a part of your regular routine. Consider a weekly brain dump to prep for the week ahead, or every night to clear your mind before bed, helping you to unwind and improve sleep quality. The key is consistency. The more regularly you perform brain dumps, the less mental clutter you'll accumulate, and the easier it will be to maintain focus and clarity in your daily life. Experiment with timing and frequency to find what works best for you. The beauty of this practice is that it's adaptable – it can be as long or as short as you need, as detailed or as brief as you want, making it a perfect fit for the variable nature of ADHD.

By incorporating the brain dump into your life, you turn a simple piece of paper into a powerful tool for mental clarity and focus. It's about giving yourself permission to unload, sort, and organize your thoughts in a way that enhances your productivity and peace of mind.

CHAPTER 19

MEAL PLANNING AND GROCERY SHOPPING SIMPLIFIED

Sometimes I'm so ADHD that I literally forget to eat. And then around 10 at night I wonder "why the heck am I so hungry?" and I remember that I didn't eat any dinner. 🤔

M eal planning and grocery shopping can sometimes feel overwhelming if you have ADHD: the myriad choices, the planning required, and the sheer monotony of the task can turn what should be a straightforward activity into a weekly saga. But it doesn't have to be that way. You can transform your approach to food in a way that simplifies these tasks and injects a bit of joy and creativity into your daily grind.

First up, let's tackle meal planning. Decision fatigue is real, especially when you have ADHD. The key here is to simplify. You can start by creating a meal planning system that revolves around themes rather than specific meals. Something like 'Meat-free Monday', 'Taco Tuesday', 'Pasta Wednesday', 'Soup and Salad Thursday', 'Pizza Friday', 'Stir-fry Saturday', 'Slow-cooker Sunday' —you get the idea. This method reduces the number of decisions you need to make and still leaves room for creativity and spontaneity. You know the base, but you can play around with the ingredients, based on what's available or what you're in the mood for.

To really streamline your meal planning, consider setting aside a small chunk of time each week to brainstorm and jot down meal ideas. This can be as simple as scribbling ideas on a notepad or pinning recipes on a Pinterest board. The goal is to create a reservoir of go-to meals you can pull out each week, making the task less about scrambling for ideas and more about assembling pre-thought-out options. This approach saves time and reduces the stress of coming up with new meals each week, making your food planning sessions something to look forward to rather than dread.

Weekly Meal Planner with Suggestions for Each Day

It's a great idea to plan out your meals for the week ahead, to reduce decision fatigue and overwhelm. Here are some super-simple ideas that require minimal prep. These basic recipes are perfect for quick, easy suppers. They are healthy and nutritious, and work even if you are on a tight budget. There are enough ideas here to take you through the month. If you mix the ideas up a little, and add your own variations, you can rely on this plan throughout the whole year.

Meat-free Monday

- Veggie Fried Rice: Stir-fry some veg (can be frozen) like peas, carrots, bell peppers. Add in the pre-cooked rice, soy sauce and scrambled eggs (optional).
- Eggplant & Tomato Stew: Sauté eggplant, onion and garlic in a pot. Add diced tomatoes and chickpeas (tinned), spices like cumin and paprika, some veggie broth (stock cube). Simmer until eggplant is tender; serve with couscous or rice.
- Greek Salad with Hummus and Pitta: Toss together diced cucumber and tomatoes, chopped red onions, black olives and feta cheese with a dressing of olive oil, lemon juice, salt & pepper. Serve with warm pitta bread and hummus.
- Mushroom and spinach risotto: Sauté chopped mushrooms and spinach leaves. In a separate pan, simmer arborio rice in vegetable broth (use a stock cube) until rice is creamy and cooked through. Stir in the mushrooms and spinach and add grated parmesan cheese.

Taco Tuesday

- Chicken Tacos: Cut pre-cooked chicken breasts into thin slices, add diced onions, cilantro, taco seasoning and salsa and serve in tortillas.
- Ground Beef Tacos: Cook ground beef with taco seasoning, serve in tortillas with shredded lettuce, tomatoes, grated cheese and a dollop of sour cream.
- Roasted Vegetable Tacos: Chop up bell peppers, zucchini, red onions and toss with olive oil and cumin. Roast in the oven at 400°F (or 200°C) for 20 minutes, until cooked and slightly charred. Serve in tortillas with chopped avocado and salsa.
- Refried Bean Tacos: Heat refried beans in a pan, serve in tortillas with shredded lettuce, chopped tomatoes, grated cheese and salsa.

Pasta Wednesday

- Pasta Primavera: Mix cooked pasta with sautéed veg, e.g. zucchini, cherry tomatoes, peas, bell peppers, in olive oil and garlic powder. Top with grated cheese.
- Pesto Pasta: Cook pasta, toss in a jar of pesto sauce, add some cherry tomatoes and top with grated cheese.
- Caprese Pasta: Cook pasta, add lots of chopped tomatoes, cubed mozzarella, some torn basil leaves, olive oil and a splash of balsamic vinegar.
- Spaghetti Carbonara: Cook spaghetti. In a pan, sauté bacon or pancetta cubes with chopped garlic until brown and crispy. Whisk up 1 egg per person and add a good amount of grated parmesan cheese. Toss hot spaghetti with pancetta, eggs and cheese until creamy.

Soup and Salad Thursday

- Italian Sausage Soup: Sauté sliced sausage, chopped onions and garlic in a pot, add chicken broth, diced tinned tomatoes and tinned white beans, simmer for 15 minutes.
- Turkey and Rice Soup: Sauté onions, celery, carrots, garlic, add chicken broth and rice. Cook until rice is tender; add shredded cooked turkey or chicken.
- Chicken Noodle Soup: Sauté chopped onions, garlic, carrots and celery in a pot until softened. Add cooked, shredded chicken. Pour in the chicken broth (from stock cube), and add egg noodles. Simmer until noodles are tender. Season with salt and pepper.
- Ham and Potato Soup: Sauté onions and garlic in a pot until lightly browned, and add diced ham. Add chicken broth and diced potatoes. Simmer until potatoes are soft. Stir in cream right at the end.

Pizza Friday – Have a day off and order your favorite pizza!

Stir-fry Saturday

- Shrimp and Snow-pea Stir-fry: Cook shrimps until pink. Remove. Sauté snow peas, garlic and ginger. Add cooked shrimp, soy sauce and a splash of sesame oil and cook until heated through. Serve with rice or noodles.
- Chicken and Cashew Stir-fry: Sauté onions, bell peppers and garlic. Add sliced, pre-cooked chicken breast, splash with soy sauce and sesame oil and add cashew nuts. Cook until heated through and serve with rice or noodles.
- Beef and Bell Pepper Stir-fry: Sauté beef strips until browned, then remove. In the same pan, sauté chopped bell peppers and garlic. Return beef to pan, add soy sauce

and oyster sauce until cooked through. Serve with rice or noodles.

- Vegetable Stir-fry: Sauté chopped carrots, onions, bell peppers, snow-peas, sliced mushrooms in a pan with garlic, olive oil, and soy sauce. Add cashew nuts and serve with rice or noodles.

Slow-cooker Sunday

- Beef Stew: Place diced beef, chopped potatoes, onions and carrots into the slow cooker. Add minced garlic, pour over beef broth; season well; cook on high for 4-5 hours/low for 8 hours.
- Teriyaki Chicken: Place boneless chicken thighs in slow cooker with garlic and ginger, pour over the teriyaki sauce and cook on high for 3-4 hours/low for 6-7 hours.
- Honey Garlic Chicken: Place boneless chicken breasts in slow cooker. Mix together honey, soy sauce, minced garlic and ketchup in a bowl and pour over chicken. Cook on high for 3-4 hours/low for 6-7 hours.
- Marinara Meatballs: Place frozen meatballs in slow cooker and cover with a jar of Marinara sauce. Cook on high for 3-4 hours/low for 6-7 hours. Serve with spaghetti.

Efficient Grocery Shopping

Next, let's streamline the grocery shopping experience. A well-organized grocery list is your best ally here. Instead of a jumbled list of items, organize your list by category: dairy, meats, fruits, veggies, and snacks. A structured list can turn a chaotic shopping trip into a smooth sail down the aisles. Consider using a grocery list app where you can quickly check off items as you go. Here are some of the best:

1. AnyList – https://anylist.com

This is a straightforward app to use. It allows you to create multiple lists, organize items by categories and sync your lists with family and friends. It can store recipes so that you can add ingredients from a recipe to your shopping list. It can also automatically sort grocery items into store sections, making it easier to navigate the aisles.

2. Bring! – https://getbring.com

This is another very simple list app for sharing. It's particularly useful if someone else is doing the weekly shopping because you can add items to the list while they are in the store. You can also customize the list with photos, which will help you identify the exact product you want.

3. Out of Milk – https://www.outofmilk.com

This app helps you keep track of what's in your pantry, lets you create multiple shopping lists, and categorizes your groceries by aisle to save time in the supermarket. It also includes a to-do list feature for non-grocery-related tasks.

When doing a big weekly shop, timing is really important. If you can, schedule your grocery runs during off-peak hours to avoid the crowds. Less crowded stores mean fewer distractions and a quicker shopping trip. And if the thought of heading to the grocery store is just too much, there's always online grocery shopping. You can make your selections from the comfort of your home, saving time and allowing you to shop without the sensory overload of crowded supermarket aisles. Plus, it's easier to stick to your list when you've got a saved list already loaded up.

Healthy Eating and Avoiding the Junk Food Snack Trap

It's not always easy to maintain a healthy diet when you have ADHD. Impulsivity and boredom can often lead to unhealthy eating habits, especially the dreaded junk food snack for a quick dopamine hit. But with a few tricks, you can tackle these challenges head-on. For impulsivity, it's all about environment control. Keep healthy snacks visible and within easy reach, like lots of fruit in the fruit bowl. A good tip is to wash and dry all the fruit before putting it into the bowl, so that it is ready to eat and doesn't require washing first. Cereal bars and energy bites are great to have on hand. A slice of cheese or a ready-peeled hard-boiled egg make quick and easy protein snacks, and you can keep a jar of nuts and seeds on the kitchen counter that you can nibble any time. As for the unhealthy snacks – don't keep them at home at all.

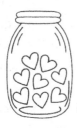

QUICK & EASY ENERGY BITES RECIPE – NO BAKING REQUIRED!

Keeping a jar or Tupperware box of these little round energy bites in the fridge can give you and your family a boost when you feel tired and tempted to reach for the junk food option. They are so easy to make, don't require any cooking and are simply irresistible.

If you have kids, you can teach them how to make these too!

Method:
 1. In a large bowl, mix together
-a cup of rolled oats,
-a cup of toasted coconut flakes,
-half a cup of flaxseeds or toasted sesame seeds,
-half a cup of creamy peanut butter,
-half a cup of honey,
-a spoonful of vanilla essence,
-a handful of dried cranberries, raisins, or chopped dried apricots.
   1. Stir everything together until it is well mixed, and chill in the refrigerator for 2 hours.
   2. Roll the mixture into 1-inch balls.
   3. They will keep in the refrigerator for around two weeks, and you can also freeze them.

HONEY

Batch Cooking and Prepping

Batch cooking can revolutionize how you handle your meals throughout the week. It's a great way of being kind to your future self. Plan on dedicating a few hours over the weekend to cook and prepare the bulk of your meals – that way, when you are tired and low on energy mid-week, you know you have something quick and easy to throw together. Here are some tips for time-saving meal prepping:

1. The Tupperware box and zip-lock bag are your best friends. Cook large portions of staples like pasta, quinoa, lentils and rice, and store them in the fridge or freezer in portion-sized containers. Don't forget to label them with the contents and the date.
2. Bake, grill, roast or sauté several portions of chicken or fish at once, and use them in different meals during the week – a batch of grilled chicken breasts can become a fahita one night, the base of a hearty salad the next night and a pizza topping the third night.
3. Keep on hand a range of different sauces and spices to add variety and flavor to your pre-cooked meats.
4. Don't be afraid to make use of frozen fruit and veg, which are pre-prepped and ready to go.
5. Trays of seasoned, roasted vegetables are so easy to cook, and will keep for several days in the fridge ready to reheat. Simply chop up whatever veg you have to hand into similar sized chunks (carrots, bell peppers, zucchini, onions, broccoli, cauliflower all go well), toss them in olive oil and throw them into the baking tray. Season with salt and pepper and roast them on a high-ish heat for around 30 minutes.

6. Batch-cook stews that are ready to reheat. One-pot meals, slow cookers, air fryers and the good old tray bake are all great ways of creating quick and easy all-in-one meals.

7. A soup maker can be a life-saver: throw in a mix of frozen veggies, a knob of butter, a stock cube and some boiling water, press 'go', and in 30 minutes, you will have a thick, hearty soup that tastes amazing. Paired with bread and a chunk of cheese, it's the perfect simple and healthy evening meal.

8. Marinate meats in a simple sauce ahead of time so that you can throw together a delicious stir-fry supper quickly and easily.

Marinating meat is a great way to simplify the prep time of your meals. You can prepare a simple marinade and keep it in a jar in the refrigerator, ready to pour over your raw meat. You can marinate meat for anything from 30 minutes to overnight, but always keep it in the refrigerator, and remember to discard any used marinade that's been in contact with raw meat.

Simple & Delicious Marinades

Here are some quick, simple and delicious home-made marinades that you can make ahead of time and store in a jar in the refrigerator ready to use:

Teriyaki – mix together soy sauce, mirin (or white wine vinegar), sugar, ginger & garlic.

Barbecue – mix together ketchup, brown sugar, vinegar, mustard, Worcestershire sauce.

Tandoori – mix together plain yoghurt, lemon juice and garlic with a tandoori spice mix.

Chimichurri – mix together parsley, cilantro, garlic, olive oil, vinegar, red pepper flakes.

Soy-ginger – mix together soy sauce, ginger, garlic, sesame oil, runny honey & rice vinegar.

Lemon-herb – mix together lemon juice, olive oil, garlic, rosemary, thyme, salt & pepper.

Spending time pre-prepping food not only saves time on daily cooking but also ensures you have healthy, home-cooked options on hand, reducing the temptation to order takeout. By simplifying meal planning, organizing your shopping, batching your cooking, and spicing up your meal routine, you can transform your approach to food into one that supports your ADHD. It's about creating systems that bring efficiency, reduce stress, and inject a bit of fun into the mundane, making healthy eating not just an aspiration but a real, achievable lifestyle.

CHAPTER 20

MAINTAINING YOUR ORGANIZED SPACE

So, let's imagine you've followed the steps in this guide and you've decluttered and cleaned your space. It looks amazing, right? You feel like a superhero who's just conquered the chaotic villain of clutter, and I hope you've given yourself a big reward. Now let's think about the next stage, maintaining the house in this state. This can be a challenge, especially when your ADHD brain is often more interested in the next exciting project than the mundane upkeep. But don't worry, you can keep your space tidy with just a small daily commitment, transforming maintenance from a dreaded chore into a quick and satisfying routine.

The Daily 5-Minute Maintenance Plan

Here's the secret to keeping your space organized without feeling overwhelmed: consistency. It's not about doing a lot at once, but doing a little every day so that the clutter doesn't have a chance to build up again. Taking just five minutes each day to tidy up ensures that you never have to face that daunting mountain of mess again. This approach not only keeps your space looking great but also gives you a sense of control and accomplishment every day, which can be incredibly motivating.

Integrating a number of mini-maintenance tasks into your daily routine ensures they become as habitual as grabbing your morning coffee. One way to do this is to anchor your new cleaning habit to an existing one. For example, while waiting for your coffee to brew, you can unload the dishwasher or tidy up the countertops. Or use the first five minutes when you get home to hang up coats and put away shoes, or clear the pet litter tray. By linking these tasks to habits you already have, you seamlessly integrate them into your daily life, making them feel less like chores and more like natural parts of your day.

Maintaining an organized space is much like gardening; it's about regular, small efforts that keep everything flourishing. Setting aside just five minutes a day for these simple tasks allows you to cultivate a living environment that remains tidy and pleasant without ever feeling burdensome. This approach makes mainte-nance manageable and embeds a sense of achievement into your everyday life, making your organized space a source of joy and pride. These small wins are also significant for the ADHD brain, which thrives on immediate rewards and success signals. Each completed mini-task is a victory, a nudge that says "hey, I can do this", boosting your confidence and inspiring you to take on the next task.

If You Do Just ONE Thing...
Top 20 Five-minute Tasks

Here's a list of 20 tasks that take just five minutes but make a huge impact. If you do just one thing today, make it one of these tasks... and don't forget to reward yourself when you're done!

1. Make the bed.
2. Clear clothes off the bedroom chair.
3. Empty the dishwasher first thing.
4. Clear and wipe down ONE kitchen countertop.
5. Sort mail and papers on the kitchen counter/table.
6. Clear out the sink, and put dishes into the dishwasher.
7. Wash up whatever is left in the sink.
8. Wipe down appliances – microwave, toaster, kettle.
9. Empty the trash and put in a fresh liner.
10. Clear and dust the coffee table.
11. Fluff cushions in living room and dust the TV.
12. Wipe down smudges & water spots in the bathroom.
13. Sort laundry into whites & coloreds, put on a wash.
14. Pick up and sort loose items on the floor of ONE room.
15. Hang up towels in the bathroom.
16. Hang up coats and jackets in the hallway.
17. Line up shoes neatly in the hallway.
18. Clean pet areas – scoop litter box, clean pet bowl.
19. Clear out and organize ONE drawer.
20. Dispose of old newspapers and magazines.

Dealing with Backsliding: Gentle Strategies for Getting Back on Track

Now let's talk about a less glamorous but utterly normal part of organizing with ADHD—backsliding. Picture this: you've spent the entire weekend getting your space just right. You've sorted, labeled, and maybe even hummed a victory tune as you admired your work. Fast forward a few weeks, and life has happened. Your desk is once again drowning in papers, and your kitchen counters are staging a hostile takeover with dishes and gadgets. It probably feels like you're back to square one. Well, here's the thing: firstly, you are not back to square one. You have already built up your cleaning and decluttering muscles, and it's not going to be hard to get going again. And secondly, backsliding isn't a failure; it's a natural part of the process. It's like being on a diet and sneaking in a midnight snack—you haven't ruined everything; you've just hit a little bump.

It's important to remind yourself that losing some organizational ground is typical. It happens to everyone, not just those with ADHD. The key is not to let this hiccup become a full-blown spiral of chaos. Instead, see it as a cue to pause and reset, rather than as a reason to criticize yourself. Cultivating a mindset of self-compassion is crucial here. When you notice the backslide, speak to yourself like you would to a dear friend—kindly, encouragingly, and without judgment, using phrases like "It's okay to hit a snag" or "Let's try this one step at a time". This gentle approach is much more motivating than harsh self-criticism, which can lead to feeling overwhelmed and stuck.

Now, on to regaining your organized state. Look back on everything we've learned, and think small—really small. The idea of reorganizing everything all over again can be daunting. But the whole point of this book is to make it easier to start a task, even when it feels overwhelming. So break it down into 5-minute micro-tasks. Can you spend just five minutes sorting today's mail? Or set a timer and see how much washing up you can do, or how much clutter you can clear off the living room floor in 5 minutes? These tiny steps are manageable and less intimidating, and they add up. You'll be surprised how quickly you can get back on track, and this can reignite your confidence and your motivation to tackle more significant tasks. Celebrate these small victories— they're important milestones on your path back to order.

Reaching out for support can also make a world of difference when you're struggling to get back on track. It could be a family member who can help sort through a pile of laundry with you, or a friend who excels in filing systems and can offer some pointers. If the backsliding feels out of control, consider enlisting professional help, like a personal organizer or an ADHD coach. Sometimes, just talking about your struggles can lighten your load and provide new perspectives. Remember, seeking help is a sign of strength, not weakness. It shows a commitment to bettering your environment and, by extension, your mental well-being.

CONCLUSION

Continuous Growth – The Journey Beyond this Book

Well, here we are at the end of our journey together, and I hope you feel it has been helpful and enlightening. The heart of this book was never about achieving a flawless state of tidiness but about giving you the tools to make meaningful changes that enhance your daily life – one step at a time.

Let's not forget the importance of a gentle, empathetic approach to organizing. Be kind to yourself. Celebrate the days when you conquer the chaos, and reward yourself, especially on the days when moving a single plate off the kitchen counter feels like a Herculean task. Every step forward, no matter how small, is a victory.

Reflecting on your growth involves regular check-ins with yourself to acknowledge your progress and recalibrate your goals. This isn't about grading yourself or focusing on what hasn't worked, but about celebrating your journey and the knowledge you've gained along the way. Regular reflection in your journal, where you jot down successes and insights, or setting aside time each week to think about what you've learned and how you've grown, solidifies your progress and enhances your self-awareness, helping you to understand more deeply how ADHD impacts your life and how you can continue to live well with it.

In wrapping up, I would love you to take away the thought that your ADHD is not a negative condition to be managed, but a dynamic aspect of your life that can enrich your experience of the world. Each step you take in learning about your ADHD, embracing change, setting new challenges, and reflecting on your growth and successes adds depth to your understanding of yourself. You're not just organizing your space or your tasks; you're organizing a life that's vibrant, fulfilling, and continuously growing. As you turn the page to the next chapter of your life, carry with you the knowledge that every day brings new opportunities to learn, grow, and redefine what it means to live your best life with ADHD.

You've got this—five minutes at a time. Here's to moving forward, embracing the chaos occasionally, and finding your own rhythm in the wonderfully messy dance of life. Keep striving, keep organizing, and most of all, keep on being your fantastic self.

* * *

REFERENCES

Online References

- *Time Perception is a Focal Symptom of Attention-Deficit/ ...* https://www. ncbi.nlm.nih.gov/pmc/articles/PMC8293837/
- *ADHD Apps: Mobile Resources for ADD Minds* https://www.additudemag. com/mobile-apps-for-adhd-minds/
- *ADHD and Dopamine: What's the Connection?* https://www.healthline. com/health/adhd/adhd-dopamine
- *ADHD Personal Stories: Real-Life Success ... - ADDitude* https://www. additudemag.com/adhd-personal-stories-real-life-people-living-with-adhd/
- *How to Get Organized with Adult ADHD* https://www.additudemag.com/ how-to-get-organized-with-adhd/
- *Stop ADHD Procrastination: Getting Things Done - ADDitude* https://www. additudemag.com/stop-adhd-procrastination/
- *Time Management Skills for ADHD Brains: Practical Advice* https://www. additudemag.com/time-management-skills-adhd-brain/
- *ADHD Bedtime Routine: How To Create One You Don't Hate* https:// blackgirllostkeys.com/adhd/adhd-bedtime-routine-how-to-create-one-you-dont-hate/
- *18 Five-Minute Decluttering Tips to Start Conquering Your Mess* https:// addfreesources.net/18-five-minute-decluttering-tips/
- *Organization Tips for Home: Clutter, Money, Meals & More* https://www. additudemag.com/category/manage-adhd-life/home-organization/
- *How to Build and Maintain New Habits* https://chadd.org/adhd-news/ adhd-news-adults/how-to-build-and-maintain-new-habits/
- *ADHD Executive Dysfunction: How to Achieve Productivity ...* https://www. additudemag.com/adhd-executive-dysfunction-how-to-be-more-productive-consistent/
- *How to Declutter: 7 Tips for ADHD Adults* https://www.additudemag.com/ slideshows/how-to-declutter-adhd/
- *Time Management Skills for ADHD Brains: Practical Advice* https://www. additudemag.com/time-management-skills-adhd-brain/

- *14 meal planning tips for ADHD brains (and why you should ...* https://www. getinflow.io/post/meal-planning-tips-for-adhd-adults#:
- *ADHD Stress Management and Coping Skills: Self-Care ...* https://www. additudemag.com/slideshows/adhd-stress-management-skills-for-adults/
- *The Power of a Brain Dump: How to Untangle Your ADHD Mind* https:// www.neverdefeatedcoaching.net/the-power-of-a-brain-dump-how-to-untangle-your-adhd-mind/
- *8 ADHD Meditation & Mindfulness Tips - Healthline* https://www. healthline.com/health/adhd/adhd-meditation
- *Hyperfocus: How to Control Your ADHD Focus* https://www.additudemag. com/slideshows/hyperfocus-for-productivity/
- *38 ADHD Home Organization Ideas, Tips, Systems & Hacks* https://www. minimizemymess.com/blog/adhd-home-organization-hacks
- *undefined* undefined
- *Best Productivity Apps for Adults with ADHD: Our Top Picks* https://www. additudemag.com/best-productivity-apps-adhd-adults/
- *Navigating ADHD @ Work - Supernormal* https://supernormal.com/blog/ navigating-adhd-workplace
- *How to Get Organized with Adult ADHD* https://www.additudemag.com/ how-to-get-organized-with-adhd/
- *Daily Routine Troubleshooting for ADHD Brains* https://www.additudemag. com/how-to-stick-to-a-routine-adhd/
- *Decluttering With ADHD: 9 Tips to Help Clear Clutter* https:// balancethroughsimplicity.com/decluttering-with-adhd/
- *ADHD Strategies: Creating Smart Systems for ADHD Brains* https://www. addept.org/living-with-adult-add-adhd/smart-systems-for-adhd-brains
- *The Creativity of ADHD* https://www.scientificamerican.com/article/the-creativity-of-adhd/
- *Marriage Communication Tips for Spouses of ADHD Adults* https://www. additudemag.com/marriage-communication-tips-adhd-spouses/
- *Your Guide to Workplace Accommodations for ADHD* https://www. healthline.com/health/adhd/workplace-accommodations-for-adhd
- *How to Set Goals and Achieve Them with ADHD* https://www.additudemag. com/how-to-set-goals-achieve-them-adhd/

General Further Reading

The ADHD Effect on Marriage – Understand and Rebuild your Relationship in 6 Steps, by Melissa Orlov, 2010

How to Keep House while Drowning – A Gentle Approach to Cleaning and Organizing, by K.C. Davis, 2022.

The Life-Changing Magic of Decluttering: A Simple, Effective Way to Banish Clutter Forever, by Marie Kondo, 2014.

How to Manage your Home Without Losing Your Mind – Dealing with your House's Dirty Little Secrets, by Dana K. White, 2016.

Decluttering at the Speed of Life – Winning your Never-ending Battle with Stuff, by Dana K. White, 2018

Organizing Solutions for people with ADHD – Tips and Tools to Help you Take Charge of Your Life and Get Organized, by Susan C. Pinsky, 3rd Edition, 2023.

Blogs and Websites

ADDitude – www.additudemag.com
This is one of the most comprehensive resources for ADHD. It offers a wealth of articles, personal stories and expert tips on managing ADHD in adulthood.

How to ADHD – https://howtoadhd.com
A blog from actress Jessica McCabe that also includes a YouTube channel, providing engaging and informative content tailored specifically for ADHD adults.

ADD Consults – https://addconsults.com
Founder of ADD Consults Terry Matlen, is a psychotherapist, writer, and certified ADHD coach, with a special focus on adult women with ADHD. This blog is packed with useful resources.

The ADHD Homestead – https://adhdhomestead.net
Author and blogger Jaclyn Paul's site is full of practical tips and personal anecdotes on living with ADHD, focusing on daily management strategies and long-term planning.

Untapped Brilliance – https://untappedbrilliance.com
This blog has been named 'Best ADHD blog' for 5 years in a row. Former nurse turned ADHD coach and blogger Jacqueline Sinfield helps adults with ADHD make sense of their diagnosis. Her site is full of resources and great articles.

ADHD Rollercoaster – https://adhdrollercoaster.org
Gina Pera's honest, no-nonsense blog covers a huge number of important issues, from nutrition to relationships, helping you to ride the ADHD rollercoaster 'without getting whiplash'.

ADHD Essentials - www.ADHDessentials.com.

Psychologist Brendan Mahan M.Ed., M.S. developed the ADHD Essentials website as a resource to help people with ADHD develop the skills and knowledge they need to thrive with ADHD. He also runs a regular podcast, with in-depth interviews with parents, educators and experts, plus a flourishing Facebook group.

Minimize my Mess - https://www.minimizemymess.com

Lots of tips and a great blog from minimalism expert Ema Hidlebaugh, who specializes in creating a more minimalist home and a capsule wardrobe, helping people with advice that is relatable and practical.

ADHD & Marriage – http://adhdandmarriage.com

Melissa Orlov and Dr Ned Hallowell blog about marriage when one or both spouses have ADHD. The website is full of insights and tips, and they have written two books: *The ADHD Effect on Marriage* and *The Couples' Guide to Thriving with ADHD*. They also run seminars and training sessions.

About the Author

Caroline Singer MA is a published author and certified ADHD coach, with a particular interest in neurodiversity and family issues. Several of her family members have ADHD, so she understands at close range what the key issues are. Her work is fueled by a passion for providing empathetic support, practical advice and uplifting encouragement. Caroline's mission is to help individuals and families living with ADHD to give themselves the gift of a calmer and more organized environment, fostering hope and positive change in their lives.

A Final Note from the Author

Dear Reader,

Thank you for taking the time to read my book. Your support and feedback mean the world to me. If you found value in this book, I kindly ask you to share your thoughts by leaving a review on Amazon. Your review not only helps other readers discover the book, but also allows me to continue writing and sharing content that can make a difference.

Thank you with all my heart for your support!

Made in the USA
Monee, IL
14 May 2025

17476155R00085